SIMPLIFIED ANATOMY AND PHYSIOLOGY
for Paramedical Students

SIMPLIFIED ANATOMY AND PHYSIOLOGY
for Paramedical Students

Manju Chhugani MSc Nursing PhD

The International Marie Goubran Agent of Change Award Winner, 2020
Dean and Professor of Nursing
Head, Department of Paramedical Sciences
School of Nursing Sciences and Allied Health
Jamia Hamdard
Hamdard Nagar, New Delhi, India

Preysi Chauhan MSc Nursing (AIIMS)

Madhav Das Bijlani Award Winner for Topper in
Anatomy and Physiology, 2013
Tutor
School of Nursing Sciences and Allied Health
Jamia Hamdard
Hamdard Nagar, New Delhi, India

Foreword
Suresh K Sharma

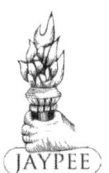

JAYPEE BROTHERS MEDICAL PUBLISHERS
The Health Sciences Publisher
New Delhi | London

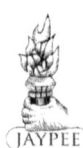 **Jaypee Brothers Medical Publishers (P) Ltd**

Headquarters
Jaypee Brothers Medical Publishers (P) Ltd
EMCA House
23/23-B, Ansari Road, Daryaganj
New Delhi - 110 002, India
Landline: +91-11-23272143, +91-11-23272703
+91-11-23282021, +91-11-23245672
Email: jaypee@jaypeebrothers.com

Corporate Office
Jaypee Brothers Medical Publishers (P) Ltd
4838/24, Ansari Road, Daryaganj
New Delhi 110 002, India
Phone: +91-11-43574357
Fax: +91-11-43574314
Email: jaypee@jaypeebrothers.com

Overseas Office
J.P. Medical Ltd
83 Victoria Street, London
SW1H 0HW (UK)
Phone: +44 20 3170 8910
Fax: +44 (0)20 3008 6180
Email: info@jpmedpub.com

Website: www.jaypeebrothers.com
Website: www.jaypeedigital.com

© 2023, Jaypee Brothers Medical Publishers (P) Ltd

The views and opinions expressed in this book are solely those of the original contributor(s)/author(s) and do not necessarily represent those of editor(s) and publisher of the book.

All rights reserved. No part of this publication may be reproduced, stored or transmitted in any form or by any means, electronic, mechanical, photocopying, recording or otherwise, without the prior permission in writing of the publishers.

All brand names and product names used in this book are trade names, service marks, trademarks or registered trademarks of their respective owners. The publisher is not associated with any product or vendor mentioned in this book.

Medical knowledge and practice change constantly. This book is designed to provide accurate, authoritative information about the subject matter in question. However, readers are advised to check the most current information available on procedures included and check information from the manufacturer of each product to be administered, to verify the recommended dose, formula, method and duration of administration, adverse effects and contraindications. It is the responsibility of the practitioner to take all appropriate safety precautions. Neither the publisher nor the author(s)/editor(s) assume any liability for any injury and/or damage to persons or property arising from or related to use of material in this book.

This book is sold on the understanding that the publisher is not engaged in providing professional medical services. If such advice or services are required, the services of a competent medical professional should be sought.

Every effort has been made where necessary to contact holders of copyright to obtain permission to reproduce copyright material. If any have been inadvertently overlooked, the publisher will be pleased to make the necessary arrangements at the first opportunity.

Inquiries for bulk sales may be solicited at: jaypee@jaypeebrothers.com

Simplified Anatomy and Physiology for Paramedical Students

First Edition: **2023**

ISBN: 978-93-5465-780-1

Contributors

Babita Bisht
Tutor
School of Nursing Sciences and Allied Health
Jamia Hamdard
Hamdard Nagar, New Delhi, India

Deepali Gupta
Tutor
School of Nursing Sciences and Allied Health
Jamia Hamdard
Hamdard Nagar, New Delhi, India

Parveen Naaz
Assistant Professor
School of Nursing Sciences and Allied Health
Jamia Hamdard
Hamdard Nagar, New Delhi, India

Vibha Kumari
Assistant Professor
School of Nursing Sciences and Allied Health
Jamia Hamdard
Hamdard Nagar, New Delhi, India

Reviewers

Paramita Deb
Assistant Professor
Department of Allied Health Sciences
Program of Optometry
Brainware University
Kolkata, West Bengal, India

Rakesh Kumar Yadav
Head, Department of Optometry
Teerthanker Mahaveer University
Moradabad, Uttar Pradesh, India

Sheeba Qumar
Consultant Optometrist
Kukreja Eye Centre
New Delhi, India

Vikas Shrivastava
Head, Department of Optometry
Program Chair, Division of Optometry
Department of Paramedical and Allied Sciences
School of Medical and Allied Sciences
Galgotias University
Greater Naida, Uttar Pradesh, India

Foreword

Generally, students opt for medical, rehabilitation, pharmacy and nursing fields, paramedical courses remain the other choice for most of the students who seek their career in medical profession. Paramedical courses are specializing in healthcare services and is suitable for candidates aspiring to pursue a career in medicine in a short duration and in low budget.

The anatomy and physiology are the backbone of general foundation course (GFC) for all health-related programs as understanding of human body, the interaction of organs with each other is crucial in medical field.

The *Simplified Anatomy and Physiology for Paramedical Students* by Dr Manju Chhugani and Ms Preysi Chauhan is an effort towards introducing an easy-to-understand book for paramedical students. The book is easy-to-comprehend and written in very simple and easy-to-understand language. It has objective type questions, short answer practice questions at the end of each chapter to aid the readers to review his learning after reading. The glossary and summary in the end help the readers to grasp maximum from the book.

I found this book suitable for paramedical students, teachers and I am confident that book will meet the expectations of readers.

Suresh K Sharma PhD RN FNRS
Professor and Principal
College of Nursing
All India Institute of Medical Sciences
Jodhpur, Rajasthan, India
ICN-Global Nursing Leadership Fellow – 2020, GNLI, Geneva, Switzerland

Preface

Anatomy is study of the structure of the body; it deals with the position and structure of organs like the bones, muscles and glands.

Physiology is the study of how the human body works; it is a subdivision of biology focusing on the physical and chemical processes of the body. From cells to organ systems, physiology is a discipline that tries to understand what happens in a healthy body and what goes wrong in these cells and systems when someone falls ill.

While these two fields may be separated system-wise for easier understanding but in practical application, the reader must remember that they all go hand-in-hand. All processes and structures are interlinked; cooperating to maintain the health of the organism.

There is no easy-to-understood book for anatomy and physiology till now and this is a general foundation course for all streams of paramedical studies.

Simplified Anatomy and Physiology for Paramedical Students is a textbook specifically designed to make this foundation course easier.

Currently, the paramedical profession is in its budding stage and there are not many experts in this discipline. This textbook has many unique features which will make it simpler for the reader to grasp concepts, such as simple language for easy understanding, designed according to the paramedical course curriculum, practice diagrams and exercises at the end of each chapter and use of labeled and colored diagrams for easy understanding of concepts regarding anatomy and physiology.

Paramedical and allied health students will find this textbook extremely helpful because anatomy and physiology are the basics of the basics that they must have a firm grasp over if they wish to excel in the field of paramedical studies.

Manju Chhugani
Preysi Chauhan

Contents

1. **Introduction to Anatomy and Physiology** 1
   - Anatomy   1
   - Physiology   2

2. **Basic Unit of Life: Cell** 6
   - Cell   6
   - Transportation Across Cells   8
   - Tissues   9

3. **Musculoskeletal System: Bones and Muscles** 16
   - The Muscular System   16
   - The Skeletal System   22

4. **Introduction to Cardiovascular System: Blood** 34
   - Composition of Blood   34
   - Functions of Blood   35
   - Cellular Elements of the Blood   36
   - Blood Group   40
   - Disorders of Blood   41

5. **Cardiovascular System: Heart** 49
   - Heart   49

6. **Respiratory System** 60
   - Functions of Respiratory System   65
   - Physiology of Respiration   65
   - Alterations in Respiration   66
   - Exchange of Oxygen and Carbon Dioxide   67
   - Regulation of the Respiratory Center   68

7. **Digestive System** 70
   - Basic Processes of Digestion   71
   - Layers of GI Tract   71
   - Mouth   72
   - Esophagus   76
   - Stomach   77
   - Pancreas   78
   - Liver   80
   - Gallbladder   81
   - Small Intestine   82
   - Large Intestine   83
   - Physiology of Digestion   85

8. **Excretory System** 88
   - Excretion   88
   - Human Excretory System   88
   - Mechanism of Urine Formation   92
   - Regulation of Kidney Function   93

- Role of Other Organs in Excretion 96
- Disorders of the Excretory System 96
- Excretion and its Importance 97

9. Nervous System 100
- Nervous System 100
- Central Nervous System 100
- Peripheral Nervous System 107
- Autonomic Nervous System 108
- Nerve Tissue 109

10. Sense Organs 114
- What are the Sense Organs? 115
- Five Sense Organs 116
- Other Sensory Organs 118

11. Endocrine System 121
- Pituitary Gland 122
- Thyroid Gland 123
- Parathyroid Gland 124
- Adrenal or Suprarenal Glands 124
- Pancreas 126
- Ovaries and Testes (Gonads) 127
- Thymus 127
- Pineal Gland 127
- Endocrine System Disorders 127

12. Reproductive System 138
- Male Reproductive System 138
- Female Reproductive System 141
- Menstrual Cycle 145
- Reproductive System Disorders 147

Index *151*

Syllabus

FC-101, HUMAN ANATOMY

Theory

Maximum Marks: 100 (75 + 25)

Unit-I
- **Introduction to anatomy:**
  - Anatomical terms, planes, organization of human body—cell, tissue, organ and organ system
  - Musculoskeletal system
  - Types of bones, structure and divisions of the skeleton system, name of all the bones and their parts, joints
  - Classification
  - Structure and types of muscles
- **Anatomy of the nervous system:**
  - Central nervous system and peripheral nervous system—different components

Unit-II
- **Anatomy of circulatory system:**
  - General plan of circulatory system and its components
  - Heart—size, location, coverings, chambers, blood supply, nerve supply, the blood vessels
  - General plan of circulation, pulmonary circulation
  - Name of arteries and veins and their positions
  - Lymphatic system—general plan
- **Anatomy of the respiratory system:**
  - Organs of respiratory system (brief knowledge of parts and position)

Unit-III
- **Anatomy of the digestive system:**
  - Anatomy of alimentary tract—parts of the tract
  - Accessory glands of digestion—pancreas, liver, gallbladder
- **Anatomy of excretory system:**
  - Kidneys—location, gross structure, excretory ducts, ureters, urinary bladder, urethra

Unit-IV
- **Reproductive system:**
  - Male reproductive system
  - Female reproductive system
- **Anatomy of the endocrine system:**
  - Name of all endocrine glands their positions, hormones and their functions—pituitary, thyroid, parathyroid, adrenal glands, gonads and islets of pancreas

GFC-103, HUMAN ANATOMY

Practical

Maximum Marks: 100 (75 + 25)

- Demonstrations of different parts of human body
- General slides of tissues and organs
- Preservation, embalming of body parts

GFC-102, PHYSIOLOGY

Maximum Marks: 100 (75 + 25)

Unit-I

General physiology
- Cell—transport across cell membrane, homeostasis, resting membrane potential, action potential
- **Blood:**
  - Composition and functions of blood RBC, WBC, platelet count, hemoglobin
  - Blood groups—ABO and RH grouping homeostasis and anticoagulants

Unit-II

- **Cardiovascular system:**
  - Cardiac muscle, pacemaker and conducting tissue
  - Cardiac cycle, cardiac output, heart rate, ECG, arterial blood pressure
- **Respiratory system:** Functions of respiratory system mechanism of respiration, lung volumes and capacities

Unit-III

- **Nerve and muscle physiology:**
  - Neuron structure and properties
  - Neuromuscular junction
- **Skeletal muscle structure:** Mechanism of contraction
- **Cerebrospinal fluid (CSF):** Composition, functions and circulation
- **Central and autonomic nervous system:**
  - Organization of CNS functions of various parts of brain, in brief composition, functions and circulation of CSF
  - Differences between sympathetic and parasympathetic division

Unit-IV

- **Digestive system:**
  - Functional anatomy, organization and innervations
  - Composition and functions of all digestive juices
  - Digestion and absorption of carbohydrates, proteins and fats
- **Excretory system of kidneys:** Functions, nephron, juxtaglomerular apparatus

- **Renal circulation:**
  - Mechanism of urine formation
  - Glomerular filtration rate
- **Endocrine and reproductive systems:**
  - Endocrine glands and hormones secreted
  - Functions of reproductive system
  - Male reproductive system: Spermatogenesis, testosterone
  - Female reproductive system: Ovulation, menstrual cycle
  - Pregnancy test

GFC-104, PHYSIOLOGY PRACTICALS

Maximum Marks: 100 (75 + 25)

- Measurement of blood pressure, heart rate, pulse rate, respiratory rate, reflexes
- Hemoglobin, RBC, WBC, platelet count, blood groups—ABO and RH grouping estimation

CHAPTER 1

Introduction to Anatomy and Physiology

ANATOMY

It is the branch of science that deals with the body structure of humans, animals and other living organisms.

Branches of Human Anatomy

- **Gross anatomy:** It is the region wise study of the human body parts and organs.
- **Microscopic anatomy:** It studies the microscopic structure of biological tissues.
- **Cytology:** Branch of biology that deals with structure and function of cells.
- **Surface anatomy:** It is known as superficial anatomy, it is the study of external features of the body.
- **Radiological anatomy:** It is the study of anatomical structures through radiographic films such as X-ray.
- **Embryology:** It is the branch of science that deals with the formation, growth and development of the embryo.

Anatomical Planes (Fig. 1.1)

- **Anterior:** Front
- **Posterior:** Behind
- **Ventral:** Towards front
- **Dorsal:** Towards back
- **Proximal:** Closer towards the trunk or origin of body
- **Distal:** Away from the trunk or origin of body
- **Median:** Midline of the body
- **Lateral:** Away from median
- **Superior:** Towards the top of the head
- **Inferior:** Towards the feet

Movements of Human Body (Fig. 1.2)

- **Flexion:** It is the movement that reduces the angle between two body parts. *Example:* Bending of elbow, bending of knee.
- **Extension:** It is the movement that increases the angle between two body parts. *Example:* Extension of elbow straightens the arm.
- **Abduction:** It is the movement that occurs away from the midline. As the term suggests abducting means taking someone away.

Chapter 1: Introduction to Anatomy and Physiology

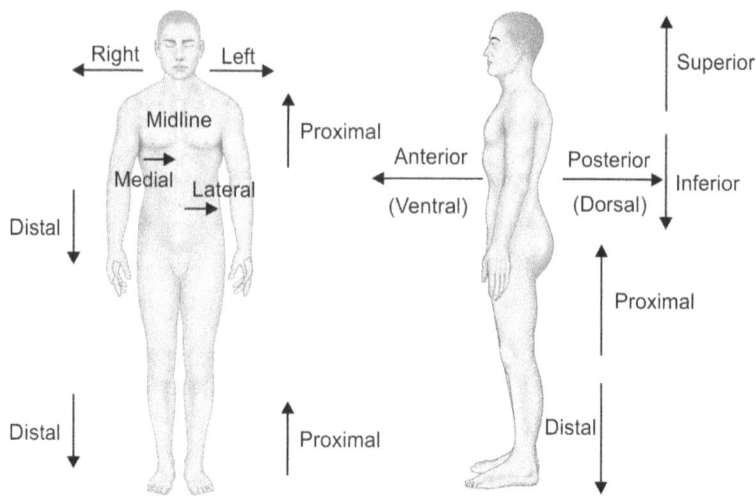

Fig. 1.1: Anatomical planes.

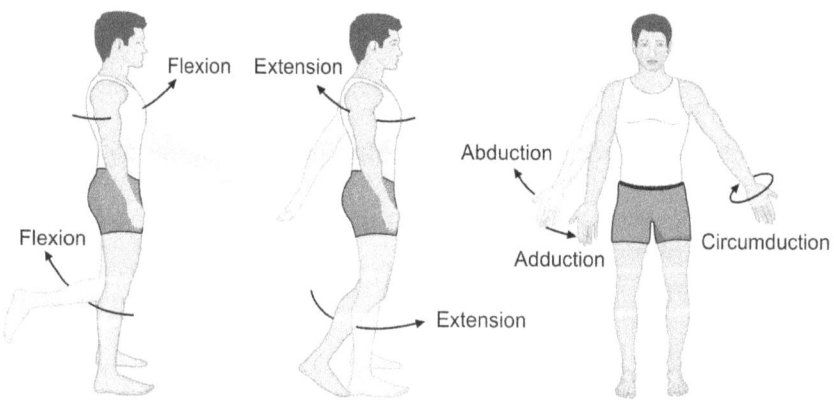

Fig. 1.2: Movements of human body.

- **Adduction:** It is the movement towards the midline. Adduction of hips puts both legs together.
- **Medial rotation:** It is the internal rotational movement towards the midline.
- **Lateral rotation:** It is the rotational movement away from the midline.
- **Elevation:** It is the movement in superior that is upper direction.
- **Depression:** It is the movement in an inferior direction.

PHYSIOLOGY

It is the branch of science/biology that deals with the mechanism or functioning of living organisms.

Chapter 1: Introduction to Anatomy and Physiology

Branches of Physiology
- **Medical physiology:** It is known as the application or use of the knowledge of human physiology to patients.
- **Animal physiology:** It is related to the functioning of animal body system.
- **Plant physiology:** It is related to the functioning of plants.
- **Cell physiology:** It is the study of functions takes place within a cell.
- **Comparative physiology:** It is the study variations of functional characteristics of different living things.
- **Cardiovascular physiology:** It is the study of functioning of blood vessels and heart.

Level of Structural Organization
- **Chemical level:** This is the basic level for the formation of body system, it includes the atoms which combines together to form molecules and they participate in chemical reactions.
- **Cellular level:** Molecules further combine together to form the cells which are the basic structural and functional unit of life
- **Tissue level:** Cells grouped together to form the tissue n they participate in specific functioning.
  Example: Cardiac tissue, nervous tissue, muscular tissue
- **Organ level:** Two different tissues combine together to form organs.
  Example: Heart, lungs, kidney.
- **System level:** Different organs combine together to form body system.
  Example: Digestive system which includes mouth, esophagus, stomach, small intestine, colon, rectum, anal canal along with accessory organs.

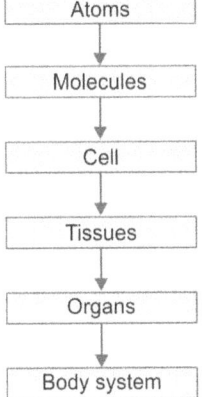

Cavities in Body (Fig. 1.3)
- **Cranial cavity:** It is formed by cranial bones and it contains the brain.
- **Vertebral canal:** It is formed by vertebral column and it contains the spinal cord.
- **Thoracic cavity:** It is formed by chest cavity that contains the pleural cavity, pericardial cavity and mediastinum.

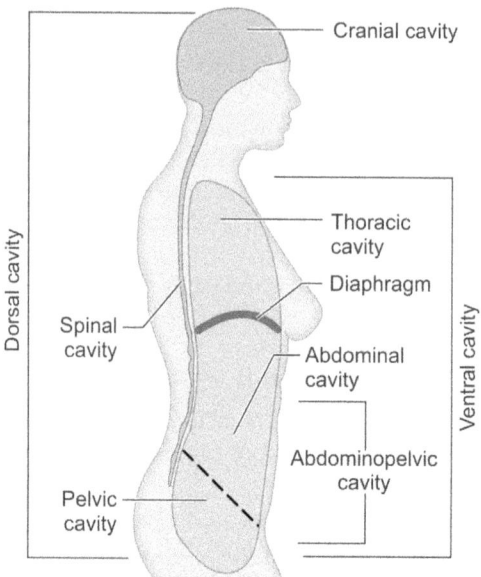

Fig. 1.3: Cavities in the body.

- ➢ *Pleural cavity:* It is the space between the pleura of lungs.
- ➢ *Pericardial cavity:* It is the space between the pericardium that surrounds the heart.
- ➢ *Mediastinum:* Central portion of the thoracic cavity between both lungs.
- ❖ **Abdominopelvic cavity:** It contains the abdominal and pelvic cavity.
  - ➢ *Abdominal cavity:* It contains the serous membrane that is known as peritoneum that surround ds the abdominal cavity along with stomach, liver, gall bladder, pancreas, small intestine and most of the large intestine.
  - ➢ *Pelvic cavity:* It contains a portion of large intestine, urinary bladder and internal reproductive organs.

Homeostasis: Homeostasis is the maintenance of stable internal environment of human body even when there is change in external environment. It is maintained through different regulatory system in body. With the changing environment, body parameters changes to maintain it normally. For instance— production of insulin by pancreas in response to the increased blood glucose/sugar level.

Hemostasis have three components to regulate body at equilibrium, they are as follows:

1. **Receptor:** There are two receptors for homeostasis that includes thermo and mechanoreceptors.
   a. *Thermoreceptor:* It is a sense receptor that regulates the body temperature.
   b. *Mechanoreceptors:* It is a sensory cell that respond to mechanical pressure.

Chapter 1: Introduction to Anatomy and Physiology

2. **Control center:** Respiratory center, renin angiotensin aldosterone system
   a. *Respiratory center:* It is responsible for maintaining the normal respiratory pattern.
   b. *Renin angiotensin aldosterone system:* That regulates the blood pressure, blood volume in body.
3. **An effector:** It is the body parts such as muscles, organ and glands that acts to bring back the body in its normal state.

Resting membrane potential: The resting membrane potential of a cell is defined as the electrical potential difference across the plasma membrane when the cell is in a non-excited state.

All cells have characteristic resting membrane potential. However, it is crucial for the proper functioning of the nervous and muscular systems.

Action potential: An action potential is a rapid rise and subsequent fall of membrane potential across a cellular membrane.

Threshold is the minimum current which is required to initiate a voltage response in a cell membrane. Stimulus current must be above threshold level to initiate response or depolarization.

Depolarization: It is activation of plasma membrane due to opening of sodium channels in the cellular membrane.

Membrane repolarization: It is coming back to resting stage results from rapid sodium channel inactivation.

CHAPTER 2

Basic Unit of Life: Cell

INTRODUCTION

This chapter is to provide an overview about the basic components of cell. All the organisms are composed of cells. The cell contains all the components and functions, which is essential for the life of the organism. Understanding the cell is crucial to understand the living being. The group of cells, which have similar structure and functions forms tissue. The organization of tissues forms the organ. The study of cell and tissue is called as cytology and histology, respectively.

CELL

Cell is the basic functional and structural unit of life. For the study purpose, we can divide it into plasma membrane, nucleus, and cytoplasm (Fig. 2.1).

- **Plasma membrane:**
  - It is the outermost protective layer.
  - It is selectively permeable
  - It acts as a barrier for different molecules and substances.

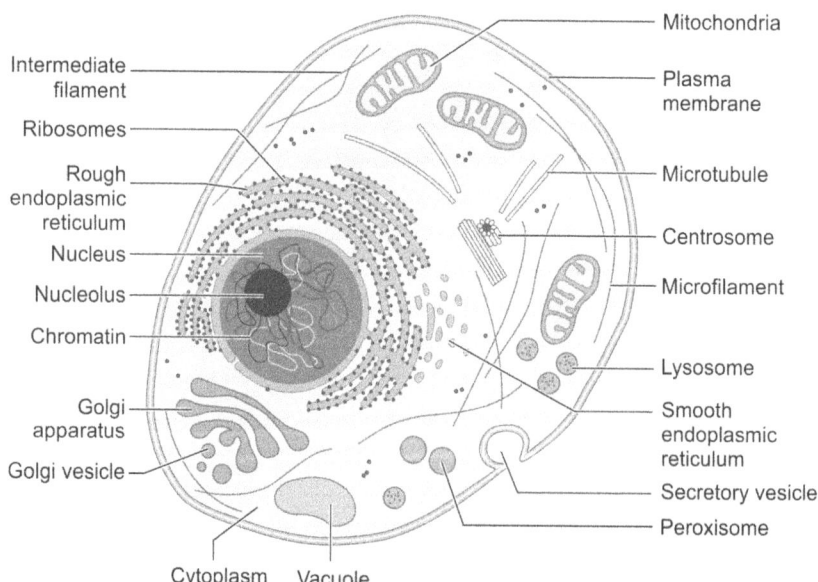

Fig. 2.1: Structure of cell.

Chapter 2: Basic Unit of Life: Cell

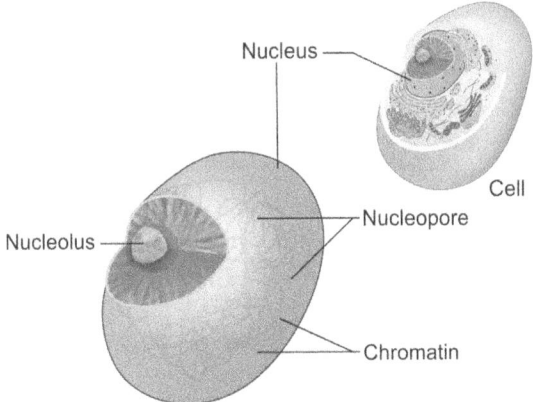

Fig. 2.2: Nucleus.

- ➢ It maintains communication between internal and external environment of cell.
- ➢ It is a lipid bilayer structure.
- ❖ **Nucleus (Fig. 2.2):**
  - ➢ It is a spherical or oval-shaped structure.
  - ➢ Its outermost layer is known as nuclear envelope, which is a bilayer.
  - ➢ Inside nucleus there are genes, which are known as hereditary unit.
  - ➢ Genes are arranged along the chromosomes, there are 46 chromosomes (each half from a parent).
  - ➢ Chromatin is the complex of DNA, RNA, and proteins.
- ❖ **Cytoplasm:** It is divided into cytosol that is the fluid portion and organelles.
  - ➢ *Cytosol:*
    - It is known as the intracellular fluid.
    - Cytosol is about 75–90% water
    - Chemical reactions occur in cytosol.
  - ➢ *Organelles:* These are the specialized structures within the cell, which have specific functions to perform and different shapes. Let us discuss all one by one.
    - Centrosome:
      - It is located near the nucleus.
      - It has centriole and pericentriolar material.
      - Centrioles are cylindrical in shape.
      - Pericentriolar material surrounds the centrioles.
      - They contain the protein tubulin, which helps in cell growth.
    - Cilia and flagella:
      - Cilia are the hair-like projections.
      - Cells of respiratory tract contain cilia, which sweeps the foreign particles away from the lungs.
      - Flagella are similar to cilia but little longer than cilia.
      - Flagella move the entire cell, for example, tail of sperm, which moves the entire sperm toward oocyte.

- Ribosomes:
  - It is the site of protein synthesis.
  - It has two subunits, one is large and other is small.
  - It is located in rough endoplasmic reticulum (ER), mitochondria, and some are located freely.
- Endoplasmic reticulum:
  - It is the network of membrane with flattened sac.
  - It is of two types rough ER and smooth ER.
  - Rough ER is studded with ribosomes, therefore synthesizes protein.
  - Smooth ER does not have ribosomes therefore does not synthesizes protein.
  - Smooth ER synthesizes the steroids and fatty acids.
- Golgi complex:
  - The synthesized protein first transported through Golgi complex.
  - Golgi complex has cisternae (cavities) that gives Golgi complex a cup-like shape.
- Lysosomes:
  - Lyso: Dissolving, somes—bodies
  - Lysosomes can engulf or eat other organelles and returns back them in cytosol for reuse.
  - The process of engulfing other organelle is known as autophagy.
- Mitochondria:
  - It is known as the power house of the cell, as they generate most of the ATP from aerobic respiration.
  - Large number of mitochondria found in active cells like muscles, liver, kidney as they uses the ATP at high rate.
  - Fluid is filled in the central cavity of mitochondria, which is known as mitochondrial matrix.
  - It also plays an important role in process of apoptosis.

TRANSPORTATION ACROSS CELLS

Transportation across the cell occurs by two methods active and passive process. Active transportations are of two types—primary and secondary, on the other hand passive process involves diffusion and osmosis. Let us discuss all processes:

1. **Passive transportation:** It is the transportation of molecules, ions across cell without the need of energy. It involves diffusion and osmosis.
   - *Diffusion:* It is the movement of solutes from their high concentration gradient to low concentration gradient across a cell without the need of energy. It is of two types, simple and facilitated diffusion.
     i. Simple diffusion: It is the process in which nonpolar molecules move across the cell without the help of transport protein and in the absence of ATP. For example, movement of oxygen, carbon dioxide, fat soluble vitamins across the cell

Chapter 2: Basic Unit of Life: Cell

    ii. Facilitated diffusion: It is the process in which the polar molecules move across the cell with the help of proteins. For example, movement of glucose across the cell with the help of glucose carrier protein.
- *Osmosis:* It is the transportation of solvent from an area of high concentration gradient to low concentration gradient across the selectively permeable membrane that is plasma membrane. For example, dialysis of kidney is an example of osmosis in which dialyzer removes the waste product from the blood via a dialyzing membrane that act as a semipermeable membrane and passes into the dialysis solution.

2. **Active transportation:** It is the process in which the molecules or substances move across the cell with the help of energy in the form of ATP. It is of two types primary active transportation in which the energy is obtained by the hydrolysis of energy and secondary active transportation.
    i. *Primary active transportation:* It involves the process of sodium/potassium pump.
        - In sodium/potassium pump three sodium moves outside the cell with the help of pump protein using ATP. In this process, three sodium molecules bind with the pump protein inside the cell, which triggers the hydrolysis of ATP and it break down into ADP and one phosphate molecule attaches with the pump protein. Protein shape changes and it pumps three sodium moves outside the cell.
        - Now the shape of pump protein completely favors the binding of two potassium molecule, therefore two potassium molecules binds with pump protein in extracellular fluid. Binding of potassium results in release of that one phosphate molecule, again the shape of pump protein changes, therefore, it results in the release of two potassium molecules inside the cell.
    ii. *Secondary active transport* refers to the use of stored ATP from primary active transportation. It involves the phagocytosis, pinocytosis, which comes under the process of endocytosis.
        - Phagocytosis is the process of engulfing foreign bodies with the help of phagocytes.
        - Pinocytosis: It is endocytosis in which the tiny droplets from extracellular space move inside the cell.

TISSUES

Cells grouped together to form the tissues. There are mainly four types of tissue, such as epithelial, connective, muscular, and nervous tissue.

Epithelial Tissue

It lines the external and internal surfaces of the body. It is of two types simple and stratified.
1. **Simple epithelium:** It is made up of single layer of epithelial tissue. It is of four types, they are as follows **(Fig. 2.3)**:

Chapter 2: Basic Unit of Life: Cell

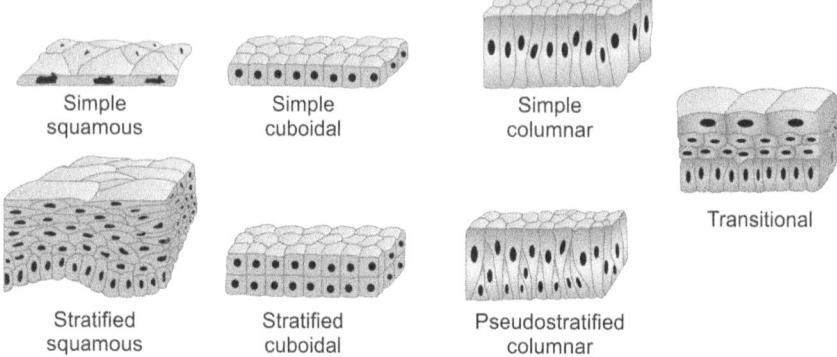

Fig. 2.3: Types of epithelium tissue.

i. *Squamous epithelium:* They have single flat layer of cells. Nucleus present in center. It lines the alveoli of lungs. It allows the rapid exchange of material.
ii. *Cuboidal epithelium:* It is the square-shaped where height and width of the cells are same. Nucleus is round and present in center. It lines the thyroid gland. It has function of secretion and absorption.
iii. *Columnar epithelium:* In this type, the height of the cell is greater than the width of the cell. The nucleus lies at the base and have elongated shape. It lines the fallopian tube, they help in absorption, secretion, and protection.
iv. *Pseudostratified epithelium:* Pseudo means false and stratified means multilayered. As the name suggests, these types of tissues shows the multiple layer of cells but in actual they have single layer of cell, due to the presence of nucleus at different level, it seems to be multilayer. They line the upper respiratory tract and helps in protection from irritants.
2. **Stratified epithelium:** It is a multilayered epithelium. It is of three types:
    i. *Transitional epithelium:* As the name suggests, they can change the shape, therefore, these type of epithelium lines the distensible organ like urinary bladder. When the bladder is filled with urine, it appears to be cuboidal-shape and when it empties it changed into squamous epithelial.
    ii. *Stratified squamous nonkeratinized epithelium:* It is a multilayered epithelium where the basal cells are columnar. It lines the epithelium lining of esophagus. It does not contain keratin, therefore keeps the area wet and moisturized.
    iii. *Stratified squamous keratinized epithelium:* It is also a multilayered epithelium where the basal cells are columnar except they contains the protein keratin, hence, it is present in epidermis of skin and protects it from UV rays, chemicals, and foreign bodies.

Chapter 2: Basic Unit of Life: Cell

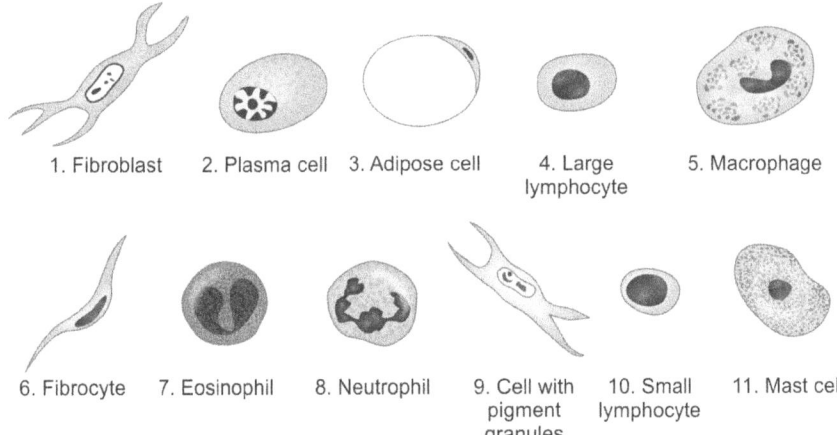

Fig. 2.4: Cells of connective tissue.

Connective Tissue

It connects the different components of body. It contains the cells, fibers, and matrix.

- **Cells of connective tissue are as follows (Fig. 2.4):**
    - *Fibroblasts:* These cells synthesis the extracellular matrix and collagen.
    - *Fibrocytes:* These are the mesenchymal cells that circulate in the blood and produce the protein such as collagen.
    - *Adipose cells:* They compose the adipose tissue and store the fat.
    - *Plasma cells:* These are the white blood cells that originate in the bone marrow and they secrete the antibodies.
    - *Mast cells:* It is a migrant cell that contains the histamine and heparin.
    - *Macrophages:* These are the specialized cells, which involves the phagocytosis.
    - *Leukocytes:* These are the white blood cells, they fight against the infection.
    - *Pigment cells:* Melanocytes are pigment cell that produces melanin and give color to the skin.
    - *Mesenchymal cells:* These are the stem cells found in bone marrow that is used for making and repairing skeletal tissues like bone and cartilage.
- **Fibers of connective tissue are as follows:**
    - *Collagen fibers:* It is a type of structural protein fiber that found in human body. It make up to 25–35% of total protein content. It is mostly found in connective tissues like tendons, ligaments, bones, skin, and cartilage. They give flexibility with great tensile strength.
    - *Elastic fibers:* These types of fibers can stretch and get back to normal size again after relieving the stretching force. These are the bundle of elastin fibers, which is produced by the fibroblasts and smooth muscle cells in arteries. It makes up to 2% of total protein in dermis. It provides elasticity and extensibility to the dermis.

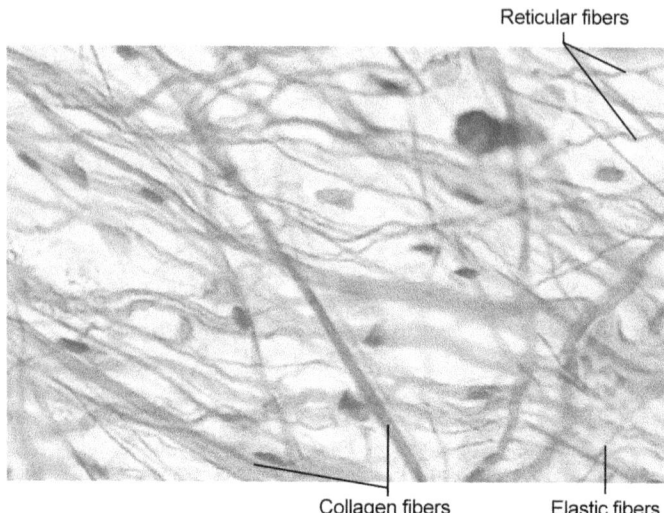

Fig. 2.5: Reticular fiber.

> *Reticular fibers:* They are the special type of collagen fibers, which is secreted by the reticular cells. They support the soft tissues such as liver and bone marrow and organs of the lymphatic system **(Fig. 2.5)**.

Types of connective tissues:
- Dense connective tissue: It is a strong fibrous tissue that makes the tendons and ligaments. Tendons connect the skeletal muscles to bones and ligaments connect bones to bones.
- Adipose connective tissue: It is a specialized connective tissue that has the lipid cell called adipocytes. They store energy in the form of fat.
- Areolar connective tissue: It is the airy (spacious) connective tissue. It surrounds the blood vessels, nerves, and muscles. It connects the skin to the underlying muscles. They hold organs in their place.
- Blood: It is considered as connective tissue as it has the matrix. It contains red blood cells (erythrocytes), white blood cells (leukocytes), the matrix (fluid portion) of blood is known as plasma.
- Cartilage: It is a type of connective tissue that have abundant amount of ground substance that gives the gel-like appearance to the tissue. It is found in joints, end of ribs, and in the vertebrae. It is of three types hyaline, fibrous, and elastic cartilage.
- Bone: It is a type of connective tissue, which have ground substance, cells, and fibers. It stores the minerals, provides strength, movements, and protects the internal organs **(Fig. 2.6)**.

Muscular Tissue

There are mainly three types of muscular tissues, they are as follows **(Fig. 2.7)**:
1. **Skeletal muscles:** They are also known as striated muscles tissue. It is under the voluntary control. It is found between bones. It helps in body

Chapter 2: Basic Unit of Life: Cell

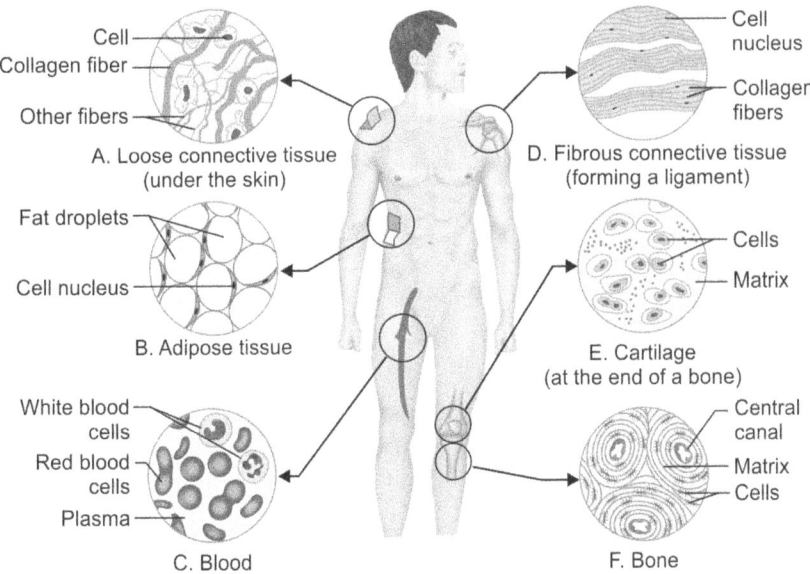

Fig. 2.6: Types of connective tissues.

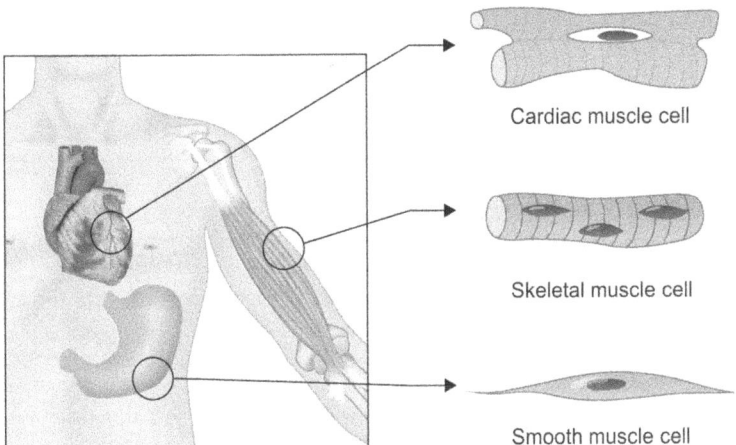

Fig. 2.7: Types of muscular tissues.

movements and to perform daily activities such as sitting, walking. They also protect vital organs.
2. **Smooth muscles:** These types of tissues are involuntary, not branched and not striated. It is located in the walls of hollow organs such as stomach and intestine. It helps in contracts, for example, pushing food forward with the help of smooth muscle tissues.
3. **Cardiac muscles:** It is found in heart. It helps in contraction of the heart to pump the blood.

Chapter 2: Basic Unit of Life: Cell

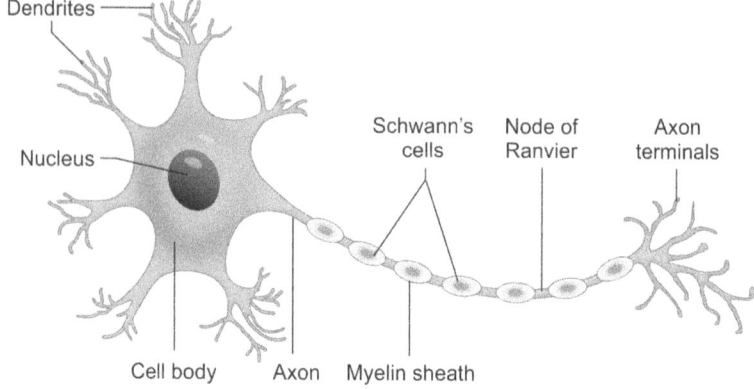

Fig. 2.8: Structure of a typical neuron.

Nervous Tissue

It is the group of organized cells that have neurons, which carries and sends the electrical signals within the body. It controls the body functions such as digestion. Nervous system is of two types, one is central nervous system that consists the brain and spinal cord and other one is peripheral nervous system that has the peripheral nerves **(Fig. 2.8)**.

SUMMARY

- Cell is the basic structural and functional unit of life.
- For the purpose of study, we divides cell into plasma membrane, nucleus, and cytoplasm.
- Transportation across cell occurs in active and passive processes.
- Diffusion is the movement of solutes from higher concentration to lower concentration across the plasma membrane.
- Osmosis is the movement of solvents from higher concentration to the lower concentration across the plasma membrane.
- Active transportation is of two types primary active and secondary active transportation.
- Tissues are the group of cells, there are four types of tissues (epithelium, connective, muscular, and nervous).

GLOSSARY

1. **DNA:** It is deoxyribonucleic acid, which is a double helix and carries genetic information.
2. **RNA:** It is ribonucleic acid which is a macromolecule. It synthesizes the proteins, and also carries the information from DNA.
3. **Apoptosis:** It is the programed cell death.
4. **Concentration gradient:** Concentration gradient occurs when concentration of particles is higher in one area as compared to others.
5. **ATP:** It is adenosine triphosphate, which is a form of energy.

Chapter 2: Basic Unit of Life: Cell

6. **ADP:** It is adenosine diphosphate, which are formed after the breakdown of ATP molecule.
7. **Liquid matrix:** It is the liquid part, for example, blood plasma.
8. **Ground substance:** It is the gel-like substance in extracellular fluid. It is mainly composed of water and glycoproteins.
9. **Dermis:** Dermis is present below the epidermis layer of skin. It has blood vessels, sweat, oil glands, and connective tissue.

LONG ANSWER TYPE QUESTIONS

1. What is cell? Briefly describe its organelles along with labeled diagram of human cell.
2. Describe active and passive transportation across the cell.
3. What is tissue? Enlists the types of tissue along with their subtypes.
4. Describe the muscular tissue and their functioning.

MULTIPLE CHOICE QUESTIONS

1. Tissues combine together to form.
   a. Body system
   b. Cell
   c. Organ
   d. Atoms
2. Power house of the cell is:
   a. Mitochondria
   b. Endoplasmic reticulum
   c. Nucleus
   d. Ribosomes
3. Sodium/potassium pump comes under:
   a. Facilitated diffusion
   b. Secondary active transportation
   c. Primary active transportation
   d. Osmosis
4. What type of muscle tissue is present in heart?
   a. Smooth muscle
   b. Skeletal muscle
   c. Cardiac muscle
   d. None of the above
5. Leukocytes is also known as:
   a. Red blood cells
   b. Plasma
   c. Platelets
   d. White blood cells

ANSWERS KEY

1. c   2. a   3. c   4. c   5. d

CHAPTER 3

Musculoskeletal System: Bones and Muscles

INTRODUCTION

Locomotor system or musculoskeletal system provides shape, structure, stability, and support to the body. It helps in the movement of the body; therefore, it is called as locomotor system. Musculoskeletal system includes bones, muscles, joints, muscles, ligaments and tendons, and soft tissues. The skeletal system includes the bones, which forms skeleton and muscular system includes muscles, which provides shape and support to the internal organs of the body. This chapter deals with musculoskeletal system and helps us to understand its structure and function.

An Overview of the Musculoskeletal System

It is subdivided into two broad systems:
1. **Muscular system:** It includes all types of muscles in the body. Skeletal muscles, in particular, are the ones that act on the body joints to produce movements. Besides muscles, the muscular system contains the tendons, which attach the muscles to the bones.
2. **Skeletal system:** Its main component is the bone. Other than its main function; the skeletal part has an important role in other homeostatic functions such as storage of minerals (e.g., calcium) and hematopoiesis, while the muscular system stores the majority of the body's carbohydrates in the form of glycogen.

THE MUSCULAR SYSTEM

There are three types of muscle tissue, based on which all the muscles are classified into three groups **(Fig. 3.1)**:
1. **Cardiac muscle:** It forms the muscular layer of the heart (myocardium).
2. **Smooth muscle:** This comprises the walls of blood vessels and hollow organs.
3. **Skeletal muscle:** This attaches to the bones and provides voluntary movement.
   The skeletal muscles are only muscles that can be controlled by the power of our will, as they are innervated by the somatic part of the nervous system. In contrast to this, the cardiac and smooth muscles are innervated by the autonomic nervous system, thus being controlled involuntarily by the autonomic center in our brain.

Skeletal Muscles

The skeletal muscles are said to be the main functional units of the muscular system. There are more than 600 muscles in the human body. The skeletal muscles of the human body are organized into four groups for every region of the body:

Chapter 3: Musculoskeletal System: Bones and Muscles

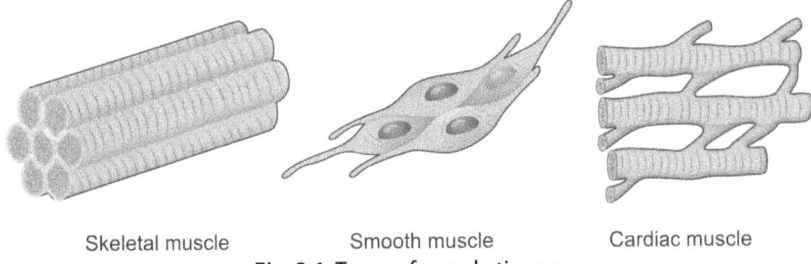

Skeletal muscle   Smooth muscle   Cardiac muscle
Fig. 3.1: Types of muscle tissues.

1. Muscles of the head and neck, which include **the muscles of the facial expression, muscles of mastication, muscles of the orbit, muscles of the tongue, and muscles of the pharynx**
2. Muscles of the trunk, which include the **muscles of the back, anterior and lateral abdominal muscles**, and **muscles of the pelvic floor**
3. Muscles of the upper limbs, which include **muscles of the shoulder, muscles of the arm, muscles of the forearm**, and muscles of the hand
4. Muscles of the lower limbs, which include **hip and thigh muscles, leg muscles**, and **foot muscles**.

Structure

Structurally, muscle fibers are specialized cells whose main feature is the ability to contract. The cytoplasm of skeletal muscle fibers (sarcoplasm), contains contractile proteins called actin and myosin.

Many muscle fibers are combined to form a group, which is called fasciculi. Each fasciculus is covered by a layer of connective tissue, which is called perimysium. Many fasciculi combine to form a muscle. Muscle is also covered by a layer of connective tissue which is called as epimysium. This layer is continuous with another—layer of connective tissue, which is known as the deep fascia of skeletal muscle that works on separating the muscles from other tissues and organs (**Fig. 3.2**).

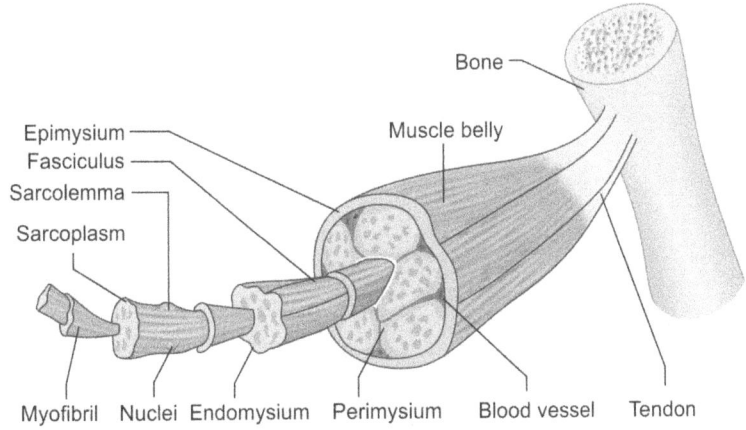

Fig. 3.2: Structure of skeletal muscle.

Chapter 3: Musculoskeletal System: Bones and Muscles

This structure gives the skeletal muscle tissue four main physiological properties:
1. **Excitability:** The ability to detect the neural stimuli (action potential)
2. **Contractibility:** The ability to contract in response to a neural stimulus
3. **Extensibility:** The ability of a muscle to be stretched without tearing
4. **Elasticity:** The ability to return to its normal shape after being extended.

Muscle Contraction

There are two types of muscle contraction:
1. **Isometric:** If the length of the muscle does not change during the contraction. For example, pushing against an immovable object.
2. **Isotonic:** If the tension remains unchanged while the length of the muscle changes. For example, walking, load is lifted.

Mechanism of Muscle Contraction

The actin and myosin filaments within the sarcomeres of muscle fibers bind to create cross-bridges and slide past one another, creating a contraction. For a contraction to occur there must first be a stimulation of the muscle in the form of an impulse (action potential) from a motor neuron (nerve that connects to muscle).

Note: One motor neuron does not stimulate the entire muscle but only a number of muscle fibers within a muscle.

❖ The individual motor neuron plus the muscle fibers it stimulates, is called a motor unit. The motor end plate (also known as the neuromuscular junction) is the junction of the motor neurons axon and the muscle fibers, it stimulates (**Fig. 3.3**).

❖ When an impulse reaches the muscle fibers of a motor unit, it stimulates a reaction in each sarcomere between the actin and myosin filaments. This reaction results in the start of a contraction and the sliding filament theory.

❖ The reaction, stimulates the "heads" on the myosin filament to reach forward, attach to the actin filament and pull actin toward the center of the sarcomere.

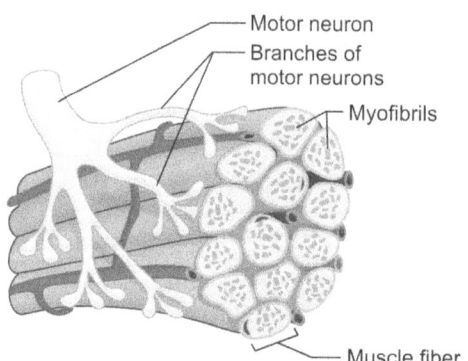

Fig. 3.3: The motor unit.

Chapter 3: Musculoskeletal System: Bones and Muscles

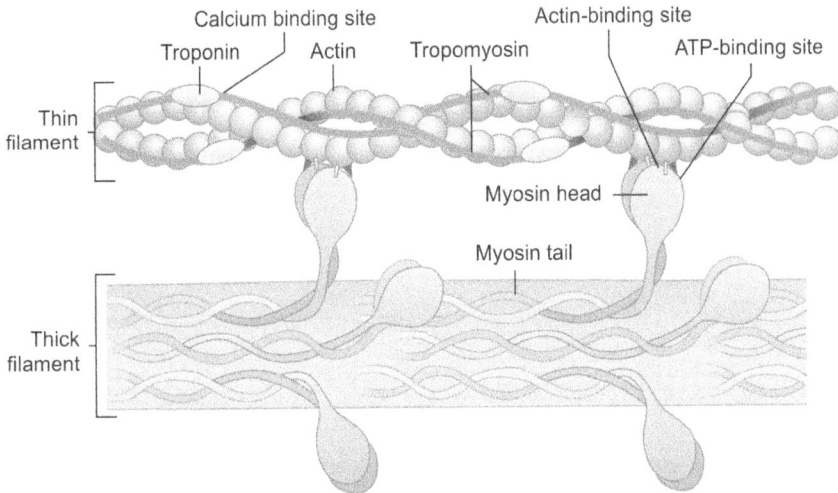

Fig. 3.4: Muscle contraction by troponin.

- Troponin is a complex of three proteins that are integral to muscle contraction. Troponin is attached to the protein tropomyosin within the actin filaments, as seen in **Figure 3.4**.
- When the muscle is stimulated to contract by the nerve impulse, calcium channels open in the sarcoplasmic reticulum (which is effectively a storage house for calcium within the muscle) and release calcium into the sarcoplasm. Some of this calcium are attached to troponin, which causes a change in the muscle cell that moves tropomyosin out of the way so the cross bridges can attach and produce muscle contraction.

In order for a skeletal muscle contraction to occur:
- There must be a neural stimulus
- There must be calcium in the muscle cells
- ATP must be available for energy

Tendon

A tendon is a tough, flexible band of connective tissue that attaches skeletal muscles to bones. Tendons are found at the distal and proximal ends of muscles, that binds them to the periosteum of bones. As muscles contract, the tendons transmit the mechanical force to the bones, pulling them, and causing movement **(Fig. 3.5)**.

Being made of dense regular connective tissue, the tendons have an abundance of parallel collagen fibers, which provide them with high tensile strength (resistance to longitudinal force).

Difference Between Skeletal, Smooth, and Cardiac Muscle

The difference between skeletal, smooth and cardiac muscles have been described in **Table 3.1**.

Chapter 3: Musculoskeletal System: Bones and Muscles

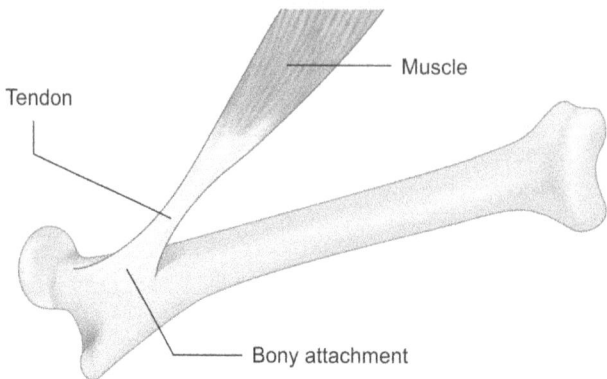

Fig. 3.5: Tendon.

TABLE 3.1: Difference between skeletal, smooth and cardiac muscles.

Skeletal (voluntary)	Smooth (involuntary)	Cardiac (involuntary)
Present in upper limb and lower limb, etc., (attached to bones and skin)	Lines walls of most of internal organs	Present in walls of heart
Controlled by central nervous system	Autonomic nervous system	Controlled by autonomic nervous system, endocrine system and various chemicals
Striated—orderly arrangement of myofibrils	Nonstriated—many myofibrils of varying length	Striated—orderly arrangement of myofibrils
Fibers unbranched	Unbranched fibers	Branched fibers
Multinucleated fibers	Uninucleated fibers	Uninucleated fibers
Oblique bridges and intercalated discs absent	Absent	Present
Cylindrical cells	Spindle shaped	Cylindrical
Blood supply abundant	Blood supply less	Rich blood supply
Fatigue easily	Does not fatigue	Does not fatigue
No rhythmic contraction	Rhythmic contraction	Rhythmic contraction

Functions of the Muscular System

The main function of the muscular system is to produce movement of the body. Some of the most important ones include:

- **Flexion and extension:** Movement of decreasing or increasing the angle between the bones involved in the movement, respectively. This motion takes place in the sagittal plane around a frontal axis. For example, **flexion** is bending the **leg** at the **knee joint**, whereas extension would be straightening knee from a flexed position.
- **Adduction and abduction:** Movements of bringing the parts of the body toward or away from the midline, respectively. For example, abduction of

the **arm** at the **shoulder joint** involves moving the arm away from the side of the body, while adduction involves bringing it back toward the body.
- **Rotation:** Movement in which a part of the body rotates around its vertical (longitudinal) axis in the transverse plane. This movement is defined relative to the midline, where internal rotation involves rotating the segment toward to the midline, while external rotation involves moving it away from the midline. For example, lateral or medial rotation of the **thigh**.
- **Supination and pronation:** These are special types of rotatory movements usually used to describe the movements of the forearm. Supination is essentially a lateral rotation of the forearm which turns the palms anteriorly (if the arm is anatomical position) or superiorly, when the elbow is flexed. These movements are also sometimes used to describe movements in the ankle and foot, in which supination means rolling the foot outward, while pronation means rolling the foot inward.
- Both during movement and stationary positions, muscles contribute to the overall support and stability of joints. Many muscles and their tendons pass over joints and thereby stabilize the articulating bones and hold them in position.
- In addition, the muscles also play an important role in maintaining posture. While the movements occur mainly due to muscles intermittently contracting and relaxing, the posture is maintained by a sustained tonic contraction of postural muscles which include the muscles of the back and abdominal muscles. These muscles act against gravity and stabilize the body during standing or walking.
- Another important function of muscles is heat production.

Positioning Terminology

Planes of the Body

Three planes of the body are used. The planes described are mutually at right angles to each other (**Fig. 3.6**):
1. **Median sagittal plane:** It divides the body into right and left halves. Any plane that is parallel to this but divides the body into unequal right and left portions is known simply as a sagittal plane or parasagittal plane.
2. **Coronal plane:** It divides the body into an anterior part and a posterior part.
3. **Transverse or axial plane:** It divides the body into a superior part and an inferior part.

This section describes how the patient is positioned.
- **Erect:** The projection is taken with the patient sitting or standing. In the erect position, the patient may be standing or sitting:
  - With the posterior aspect against the cassette
  - With the anterior aspect against the cassette
  - With the right or left side against the cassette.
- **Decubitus:** The patient is lying down. In the decubitus position, the patient may be lying in any of the following positions:
  - *Supine (dorsal decubitus):* Lying on the back.
  - *Prone (ventral decubitus):* Lying face-down.

Chapter 3: Musculoskeletal System: Bones and Muscles

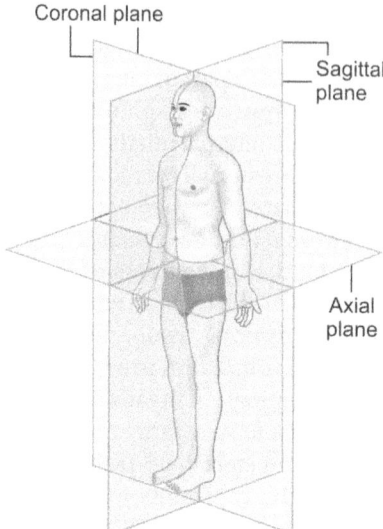

Fig. 3.6: Planes of the body.

> *Lateral decubitus:* Lying on the side.
>   - Right lateral decubitus: Lying on the right side.
>   - Left lateral decubitus: Lying on the left side.
- **Semi-recumbent:** Reclining, part way between supine and sitting erect, with the posterior aspect of the trunk against the cassette.

Terminology used: Positioning for limb radiography may include:
- A description of the aspect of the limb in contact with the cassette
- The direction of rotation of the limb in relation to the anatomical position
- The movements and degree of movement, of the various joints concerned.
- **Extension:** When the angle of the joint increases.
- **Flexion:** When the angle of the joint decreases.
- **Abduction:** Refers to a movement away from the midline.
- **Adduction:** Refers to a movement toward the midline.
- **Rotation:** Movement of the body part around its own axis, e.g., pronation: movement of the hand and forearm in which the palm is moved from facing anteriorly (as per anatomical position) to posteriorly. Supination is the reverse of this (**Fig. 3.7**).

THE SKELETAL SYSTEM

The adult human skeleton is composed of 206 bones and their associated cartilages. The bones are supported by ligaments, tendons, bursae, and muscles.

The bones of the body are grouped within the two distinct divisions:
1. **Axial skeleton:** It includes the bones along the long axis of the body. The axial skeleton consists of the **vertebral column, bones of the head**, and bones of the **thoracic cage**.

Chapter 3: Musculoskeletal System: Bones and Muscles

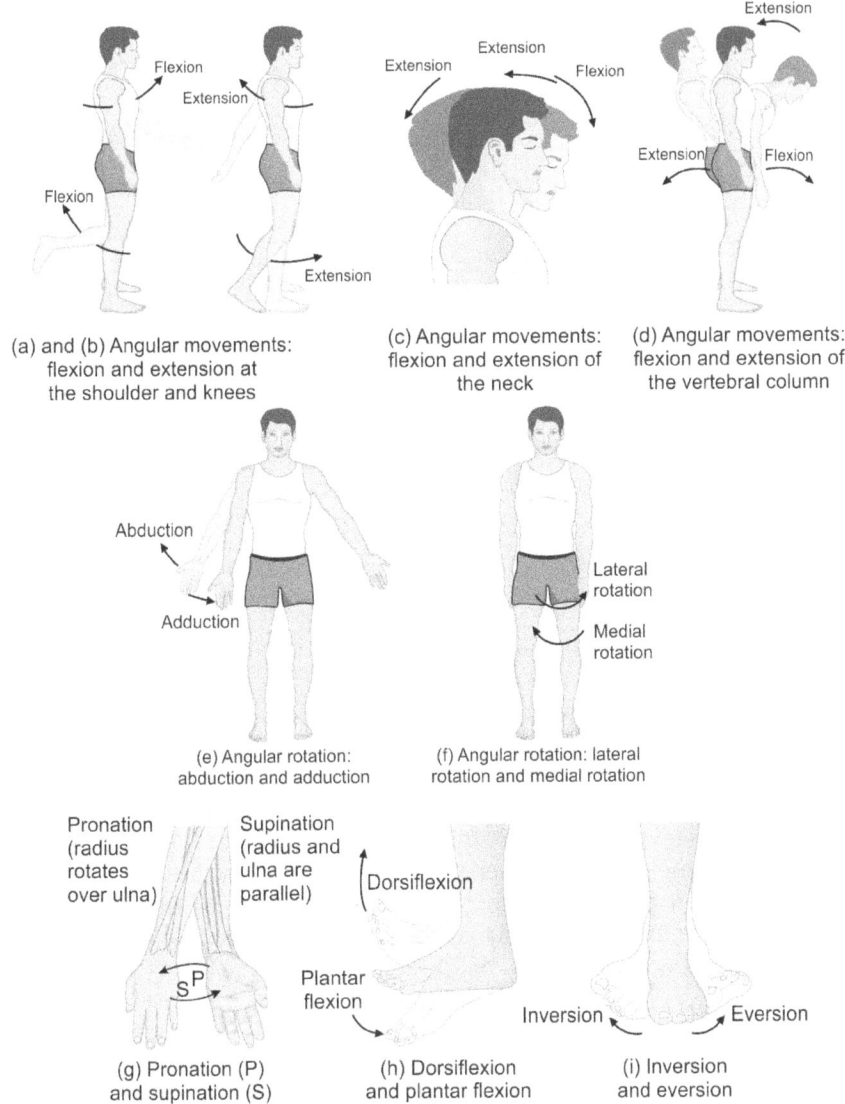

Fig. 3.7: Positioning for limb radiography.

2. **Appendicular skeleton:** It involves the bones of the shoulder and pelvic girdle, as well as the bones of the **upper** and **lower extremities**.

Axial Skeleton

The axial skeleton functions to support and protect the organs of the dorsal and ventral cavities **(Fig. 3.8)**.

The primary divisions of the skeleton system are:
- Head, including the bones of the skull (cranium), face, auditory ossicles, and hyoid bone.

Chapter 3: Musculoskeletal System: Bones and Muscles

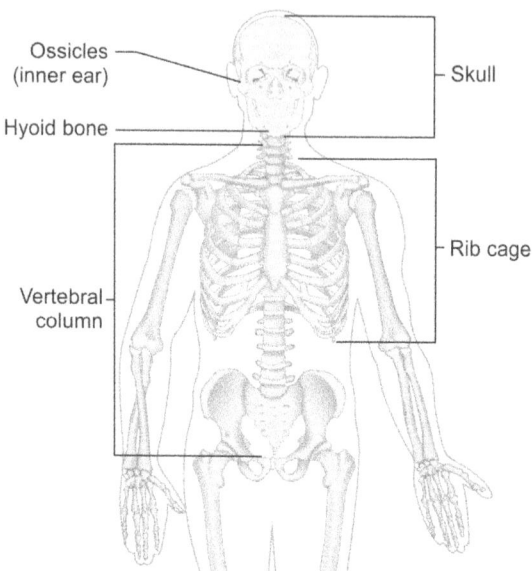

Fig. 3.8: Axial skeleton.

- Thorax, including the rib cage and sternum.
- Vertebral column.

Bones of the Head Skull (Cranium)

- The human cranium consists of the flat bones and it includes the facial bones. The cranium protects the brain
- 14 facial bones form the lower front part of the cranium.
- The immature cranium has separate plates to allow the flexibility needed for a newborn to pass through the birth canal and pelvis (**Fig. 3.9**).

These plates fuse as the skull matures (except the mandible). The human cranium supports the structures of the face and forms the brain cavity.

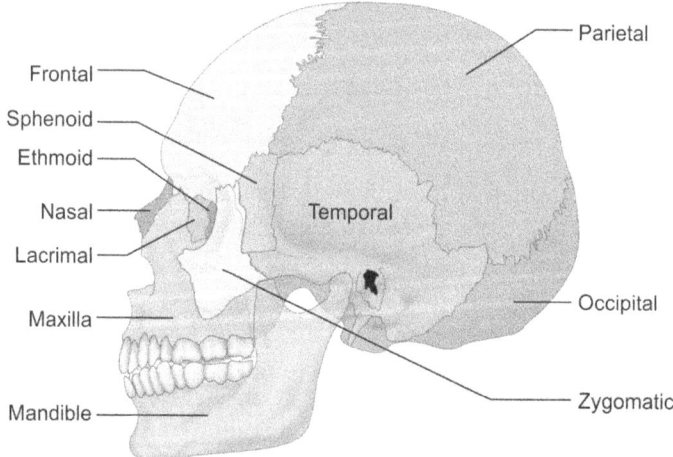

Fig. 3.9: Bones of the skull.

Chapter 3: Musculoskeletal System: Bones and Muscles

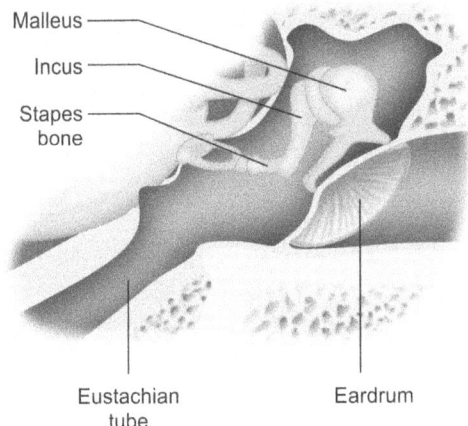

Fig. 3.10: Ossicle.

Ossicle

The ossicles (also called auditory ossicles) consist of three bones (malleus, incus, and stapes) that are the smallest in the body (**Fig. 3.10**).

Hyoid Bone

It only has muscular, ligamentous, and cartilaginous attachments.

Rib Cage

It functions as protection for the vital organs of the chest, such as the heart and lungs. The rounded ends are attached at joints to the thoracic vertebrae posteriorly and the flattened ends come together at the sternum anteriorly.

The length of each rib pair increases from number one to seven. After rib seven, the size begins to decrease. The 8th through 10th ribs have noncostal cartilage that connects them to the ribs above (**Fig. 3.11**).

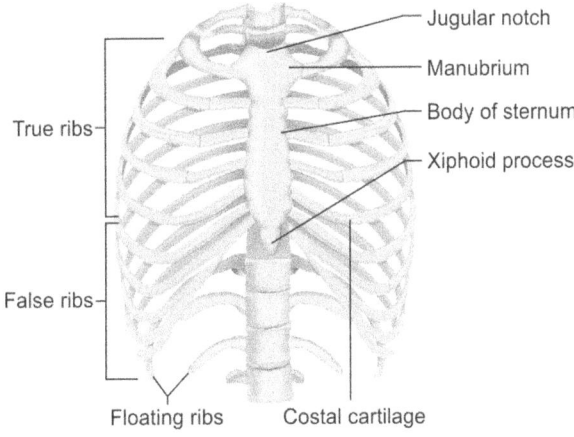

Fig. 3.11: Rib cage.

Chapter 3: Musculoskeletal System: Bones and Muscles

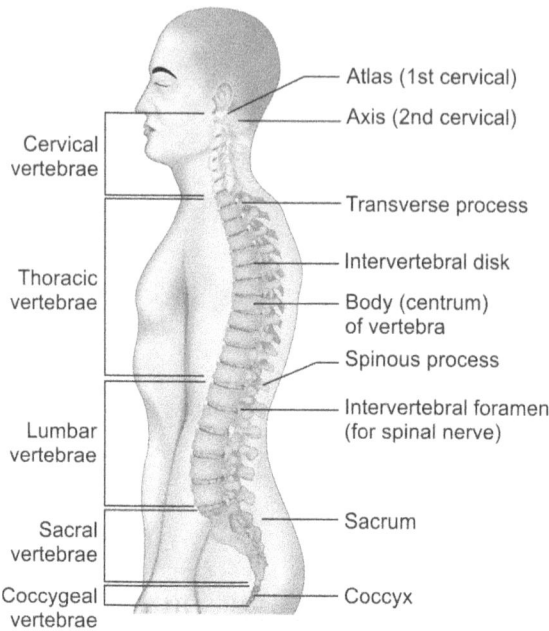

Fig. 3.12: Vertebral column.

Vertebral Column

The articulating vertebrae are named according regions:
* Cervical vertebrae (7)
* Thoracic (12)
* Lumbar (5)

The first and second cervical vertebrae are the atlas and axis, respectively, on which the head rests. The cervical vertebrae make up the junction between the vertebral column and the cranium, and the bone makes up the junction between the vertebral column and the pelvic bones (**Fig. 3.12**).

Appendicular Skeleton

The appendicular skeleton is divided into six major regions (**Fig. 3.13**):
1. The pectoral girdles consist of four bones. The left and right clavicle (2) and the scapula (2).
2. The upper arms and forearms are made up of six bones—the left and right humerus (upper arm, 2), the ulna (2), and the radius (forearm, 2).
3. The hands have 54 bones—the left and right carpals (wrist, 16), metacarpals (10), proximal phalanges (10), intermediate phalanges (8), and the distal phalanges (10).
4. The pelvis has two bones—the left and right hip bone (2).
5. The thighs and legs have 8 bones—the left and right femur (thigh, 2), patella (knee, 2), tibia (2), and fibula (leg, 2).

Chapter 3: Musculoskeletal System: Bones and Muscles

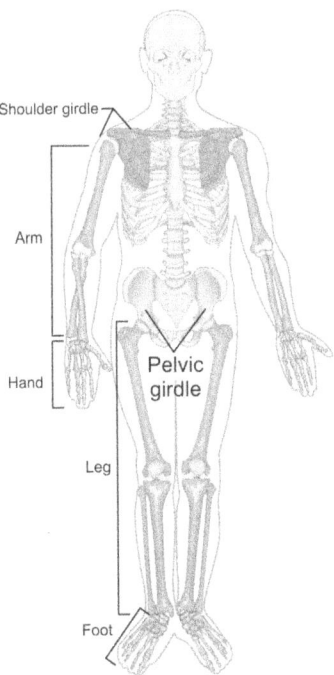

Fig. 3.13: Appendicular skeleton.

6. The feet and ankles have 52 bones—the left and right tarsals (ankle, 14), metatarsals (10), proximal phalanges (10), intermediate phalanges (8), and distal phalanges (10).

Pectoral Girdle
- The bones of the pectoral girdle consist of two bones (scapula and clavicle) and anchor the upper limb to the thoracic cage of the axial skeleton.
- The three regions of the upper limb are: arm (humerus), forearm (ulna medially and radius laterally), and the hand.
- The fingers and thumb contain a total of 14 bones, called phalanges (**Fig. 3.14**).

Pelvic Girdle
The pelvic girdle is formed by a single bone, the hip or coxal bone (also called as innominate bone), and serves as the attachment point for each lower limb.

The lower limb contains 30 bones and is divided into three regions, the thigh, leg, and foot. These consist of the femur, patella, tibia, fibula, tarsal bones, metatarsal bones, and phalanges (**Fig. 3.15**).
- The femur is the single bone of the thigh.
- The patella (kneecap) articulates with the distal femur.
- The tibia is located on the medial side of the leg
- The fibula is the thin bone of the lateral leg.
- The bones of the foot are divided into three groups, the tarsal bones, metatarsal bones, and phalanges of the foot.

Chapter 3: Musculoskeletal System: Bones and Muscles

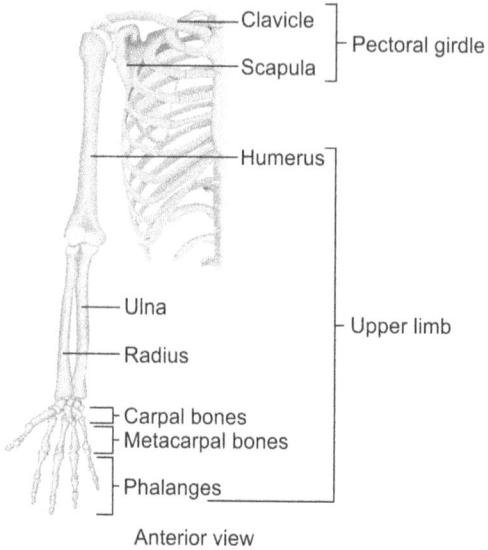

Fig. 3.14: Pectoral girdle.

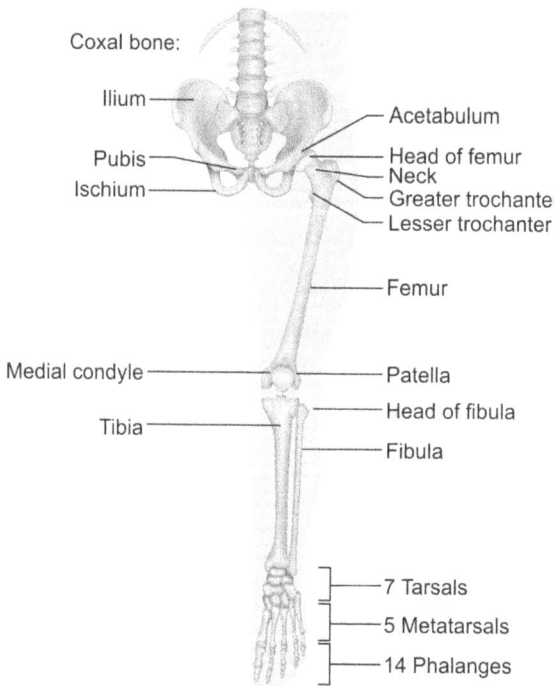

Fig. 3.15: Pelvic girdle.

Types of Bones
Bones can be classified according to their shapes as follows:
- Long bones have a tubular shape, with a longer longitudinal and a shorter transverse diameter. They are composed mostly of compact bone, while the spongy bone and bony marrow fill the ends of the bones.
  Example: Long bones include the **humerus, ulna, tibia,** and **clavicle**.
- Short bones have a roughly cuboid or round shape, and only contain a thin layer of compact bone surrounding the spongy bone.
  Example: The tarsal and **carpal bones**.
- Flat bones are mostly thin, flattened, and usually curved. They contain two parallel layers of compact bones surrounding a layer of spongy bone.
  Example: Most of the **skull bones, scapula, sternum,** and **sacrum**.
- Sesamoid bones are small, rounded unique types of bones that are embedded in muscle tendons where the tendon passes over a joint.
- Irregular bones do not fit into any of the other categories.
  Example: The **vertebrae, hip bone,** and some bones of the skull.

Cartilage
Cartilage is a flexible connective tissue found in multiple organ systems of the body. Cartilage is composed of specialized cells called chondrocytes, collagen fibers and abundant ground substance rich in proteoglycan and elastin fibers.

Cartilage is classified into the following types based on its composition:
1. **Hyaline cartilage:** Composed of type II collagen and an abundance of ground substance, which gives it a glossy appearance.
2. **Elastic cartilage:** It is similar to hyaline cartilage but contains more elastic fibers. It is found in structures such as the pinna of the **ear, auditory tube,** and **epiglottis**.
3. **Fibrocartilage:** It is composed of plenty of collagen fibers type I and a smaller amount of ground substance.
   The articular cartilage provides congruence to the articulating bones and allows them to bear weight and glide over each other with very little friction.

Joints
The integrity or stability of a joint is provided by several factors including the bony congruence and structures that cross the joint, such as tendons and ligaments.

Joints have been classified into three major structural forms, namely, fibrous, cartilaginous, and synovial:
1. **Fibrous joints** (immovable joints) (SYNARTHROSES) do not allow any movement.
   ➢ This type of joint is shown by the flat skull bones which fuse end to-end with the help of dense fibrous connective tissues in the form of sutures, to form the cranium.
2. **Cartilaginous joints** (SYNCHONDROSIS)
   ➢ The bones involved are joined together with the help of cartilages.

Chapter 3: Musculoskeletal System: Bones and Muscles

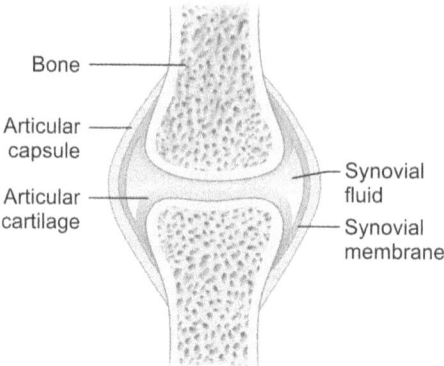

Fig. 3.16: Synovial joint.

➢ The joint between the adjacent vertebrae in the vertebral column is of the pattern and it permits limited movements.
3. Synovial joints (DIARTHROSES)
   ➢ Characterized by the presence of a fluid filled synovial cavity between the articulating surfaces of the two bones.
   ➢ This arrangement allows considerable movement. These joints help in locomotion and many other movements.
   ➢ Few examples:
     • Ball and socket joint (between humerus and pectoral girdle)
     • Hinge joint (knee joint)
     • Pivot joint (between atlas and axis)
     • Gliding joint (between the carpals)
     • Saddle joint (between carpal and metacarpal of thumb) **(Fig. 3.16)**.

Ligaments
In the musculoskeletal system, ligaments stabilize the articulating bones and reinforce the joints.

Bursae
Bursae are small sac-like outpouchings of the joint cavity lined by synovial membrane.

Functions of the Skeletal System
❖ The skeletal system serves a variety of functions.
❖ Due to its structural integrity, the skeletal system protects the internal organs, most importantly the brain, which is surrounded by the skull, as well as the heart and lungs, which are protected by the rib cage.
❖ The skeletal system also serves several metabolic functions. The bones are the storage site of important minerals, most notably calcium and phosphorus. This makes the bones essential for balancing calcium levels in the blood, which is regulated by adjusting the rate of bone resorption.

Chapter 3: Musculoskeletal System: Bones and Muscles

❖ Lastly, the bone marrow found in spongy bone is the site of **hematopoiesis**, which is a process of production of new blood cells. Cells that are produced in the bone marrow are red blood cells, platelets and white blood cells, such as monocytes, granulocytes, and lymphocytes.

SUMMARY

- The musculoskeletal system is an organ system whose primary functions include supporting the body, allowing motion, protecting vital organs, and maintaining stability during locomotion.
- It is subdivided into two broad systems—the muscular and the skeletal system.
- The skeletal muscles are the main functional units of the muscular system.
- The main function of the muscular system is to produce movement of the body. Some of the most important ones include:
  - Flexion and extension
  - Adduction and abduction
  - Rotation
  - Supination and pronation
- Both during movement and stationary positions, muscles contribute to the overall support and stability of joints. They also play an important role in maintaining posture and heat production.
- The adult human skeleton is composed of 206 bones.
- The bones of the body are grouped within the two distinct divisions—the axial and the appendicular skeleton.
- The axial skeleton consists of the **vertebral column**, **bones of the head**, and bones of the **thoracic cage**.
- The human cranium supports the structures of the face and forms the brain cavity.
- The appendicular skeleton involves the bones of the shoulder and pelvic girdle, as well as the bones of the **upper** and **lower extremities**.
- The bones of the pectoral girdle anchor the upper limb to the thoracic cage of the axial skeleton. The pelvic girdle is formed by a single bone and serves as the attachment point for each lower limb.
- According to shape, bones can be classified into the following:
  - Long bones
  - Short bones
  - Flat bones
  - Sesamoid bones
  - Irregular bones
- Each bone of the musculoskeletal system is connected to one or more bones via joints.
- Joints have been classified into three major structural forms, namely, fibrous, cartilaginous, and synovial.
- Functions of the skeletal system include:
  - Biomechanical basis of movement.
  - Protects the internal organs
  - Serves several metabolic functions.
  - Hematopoiesis

Chapter 3: Musculoskeletal System: Bones and Muscles

GLOSSARY

1. **Cardiac muscle:** Which forms the muscular layer of the heart (myocardium).
2. **Smooth muscle:** Which comprises the walls of blood vessels and hollow organs.
3. **Skeletal muscle:** Which attaches to the bones and provides voluntary movement.
4. **Isometric contraction:** If the length of the muscle does not change during the contraction.
5. **Isotonic contraction:** If the tension remains unchanged while the length of the muscle changes.
6. **Tendon:** A tendon is a tough, flexible band of connective tissue that attach skeletal muscles to bones.
7. Ligaments are elastic bands of tissue which connects bones and provide stability and strength to the joint.
8. Bursae are small sac-like outpouchings of the joint cavity lined by synovial membrane.

LONG ANSWER TYPE QUESTIONS

1. Describe the structure of skeletal muscle with diagram.
2. Explain the sliding filament theory of muscle contraction.
3. Distinguish between skeletal, smooth and cardiac muscles.
4. Classify bones according to shape and describe them with examples.
5. Write down the functions of the skeletal system.

SHORT ANSWER TYPE QUESTIONS

1. What do you understand by adduction and abduction?
2. What is a joint? Classify it according to structure.
3. Describe synovial joints.
4. Classify the bones of the skull.
5. What is a tendon?

MULTIPLE CHOICE QUESTIONS

1. Joint between bones of human skull is:
    a. Hinge joint
    b. Synovial joint
    c. Cartilaginous joint
    d. Fibrous joint
2. In humans, coccyx is formed by the fusion of vertebrae:
    a. 3
    b. 4
    c. 5
    d. 6
3. Pivot joint occurs at:
    a. The hip and shoulder joint
    b. Between the atlas and the odontoid process of the axis
    c. Sternoclavicular joint
    d. Temporomandibular joint
4. Total number of bones in appendicular skeleton of human:
    a. 126
    b. 80
    c. 44
    d. 33

Chapter 3: Musculoskeletal System: Bones and Muscles

5. Scapula is a part of:
   a. Skull
   b. Pelvic girdle
   c. Pectoral girdle
   d. Vertebral column
6. Which of the following is a sesamoid bone?
   a. Pelvic
   b. Patella
   c. Pterygoid
   d. Pectoral girdle
7. Which one is a flat bone?
   a. Scapula
   b. Carpal
   c. Patella
   d. Tarsals
8. Which of the following joints will allow no movement?
   a. Ball and socket joint
   b. Fibrous joint
   c. Cartilaginous joint
   d. Synovial joint
9. The number of floating ribs in human body:
   a. 6 pairs
   b. 5 pairs
   c. 3 pairs
   d. 2 pairs
10. Which type of muscle is controlled by both CNS and ANS?
    a. Cardiac muscle
    b. Smooth muscle
    c. Skeletal muscle
    d. None of these

ANSWERS KEY

1. d
2. c
3. b
4. a
5. c
6. b
7. a
8. b
9. d
10. a

CHAPTER 4

Introduction to Cardiovascular System: Blood

INTRODUCTION

Blood is a specialized form of connective tissue, which circulates in a closed system of blood vessels and is composed of transparent fluid plasma in which different types of cells are suspended. The concentration of plasma in blood is about 55% and cells constitute about 45% of the blood volume.

The circulating blood consists of suspension of formed elements such as erythrocytes leukocytes, and platelets in a pale-yellow colored fluid called plasma. Blood is thicker and more viscous than water. The blood is alkaline in nature and having pH of 7.4 (normal ranges 7.35–7.5). In adults, the total volume of blood comprises about 80% of the total body weight. The total blood volume in average adults is 5–6 L in males and 4–5 L in females.

The study of blood, blood forming tissues, and their associated disorders is called hematology. The word (heme) comes from the Greek for blood.

COMPOSITION OF BLOOD

Blood contains plasma (straw-colored fluid) and cells. Plasma constitutes 91% of water and dissolved substance. Dissolved substances include protein 8% and salt 0.9% **(Fig. 4.1)**.

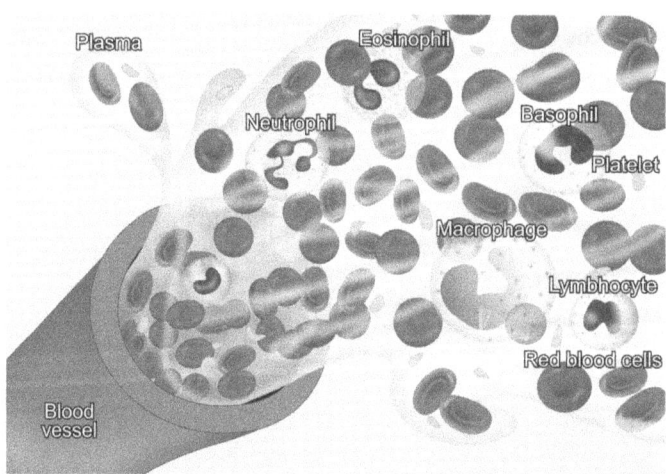

Fig. 4.1: Blood vessel containing cells.

Chapter 4: Introduction to Cardiovascular System: Blood

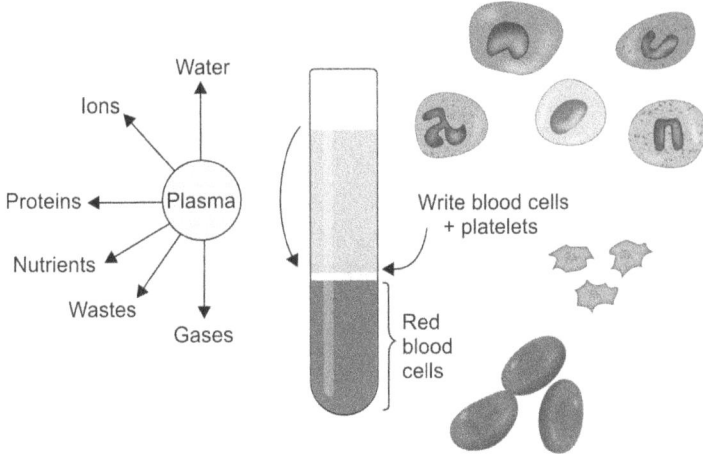

Fig. 4.2: Different cells of the blood.

Plasma contains the following (Fig. 4.2):
- **Nutrients:** Monosaccharides, amino acids, fatty acids, and vitamins from food.
- **Organic material:** Cholesterol, urea, uric acid, and creatinine.
- **Plasma proteins:** Albumin, globulin, and fibrinogen
- **Inorganic minerals:** Sodium chloride, copper, iodine, sodium, potassium, calcium, iron phosphorus, etc.
- Enzymes
- Hormones
- Antibodies
- Gases

Cellular content (formed elements) of blood contains the following:
- Leukocyte or white blood cells
- Erythrocytes or red blood cells
- Thrombocytes or platelets

The concentration of erythrocytes constitutes 95% of the cellular elements. Leukocytes and thrombocytes constitute for the remaining 5% of the volume of the cellular elements (**Figs. 4.3 and 4.4**).

FUNCTIONS OF BLOOD

- **Respiration:** Transportation of oxygen from lungs to tissues and carbon dioxide from tissues to lungs.
- **Coagulation of blood:** It contains factors of clotting mechanism, preventing blood loss from ruptured blood vessels.
- **Excretion:** Transport of metabolic wastes to the lungs, kidneys, intestine, and skin for removal.
- **Nutrition:** Transport nutrient materials such as fatty acids, monosaccharides, and amino acids from GI tract to tissues and waste materials to excretory organs such as kidneys.

Chapter 4: Introduction to Cardiovascular System: Blood

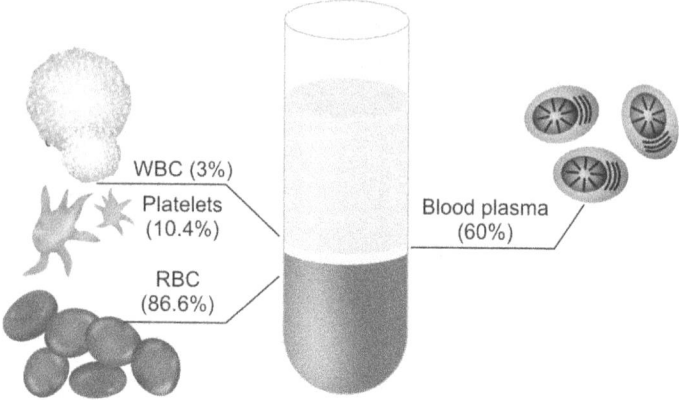

Fig. 4.3: Cellular content of blood.

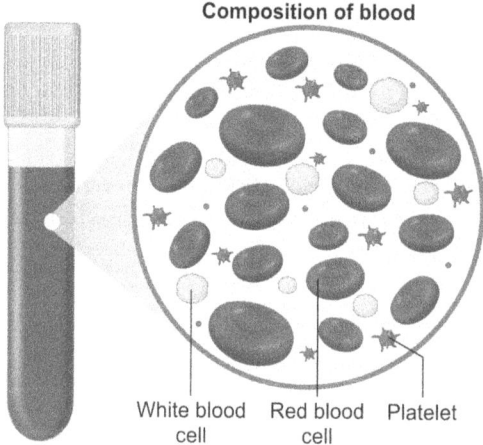

Fig. 4.4: Composition of blood.

- Transport hormones from glands to the organs.
- Maintain a normal acid-base balance of the body.
- Regulation of water balance.
- Regulation of body temperature.
- Transportation of metabolites.
- Defense against infection by the white cells and the antibodies.

CELLULAR ELEMENTS OF THE BLOOD

Red Blood Corpuscles (RBC) or Erythrocytes

Erythrocytes (**erythros: red and cytos: cell**) are the most numerous of the blood elements that have been formed. They are non-nucleated cells that are spherical, biconcave, disc shaped. RBC contains a pigment of hemoglobin that is able to bind with oxygen and release it during its circulation to the tissues of the body. Carbon dioxide is then absorbed by the red cells from the tissues

Chapter 4: Introduction to Cardiovascular System: Blood

and taken to the lungs to be exhaled. The standard range is between 4 and 5.5 lakhs per cubic millimeter.

Red blood cells are produced in the long bones, flat, and irregular bones of the red bone marrow. RBCs' lifetime is roughly 120 days.

Erythropoiesis

The process of development of RBCs is called erythropoiesis. According to the monophyletic theory, the various cells concerned in normoblasts erythropoiesis are hemocytoblast, proerythroblast, early normoblast, intermediate normoblast, late normoblast, reticulocyte, and mature RBC.

- **Hemocytoblast:** A large cell with a diameter of 18-24 microns, two or more nucleoli and agranular cytoplasm.
- **Proerythroblast:** Agranular cytoplasm, 14-19 microns in diameter, large round nucleus.
- **Early normoblast:** Agranular cytoplasm 11-17 microns in diameter, large nucleus but without nucleoli,
- **Intermediate normoblast:** Cell with diameter of 10-14 microns, nucleus smaller than that of the precursor, bluish red cytoplasm.
- **Late normoblast:** Cell with diameter of 7-10 microns, red cytoplasm (fully hemoglobinized)
- **Reticulocyte:** A non-nucleated cell, the size of a mature or slightly larger erythrocyte.
- **Mature erythrocyte:** Non-nucleated 7.2 microns in diameter, biconcave disc, cytoplasm uniformly red with a faint central Pallor (**Fig. 4.5**).

Hemoglobin

Hemoglobin is a conjugated protein that acts as a vehicle for oxygen and carbon dioxide transport. It is composed of four protein chains, two alpha chains and

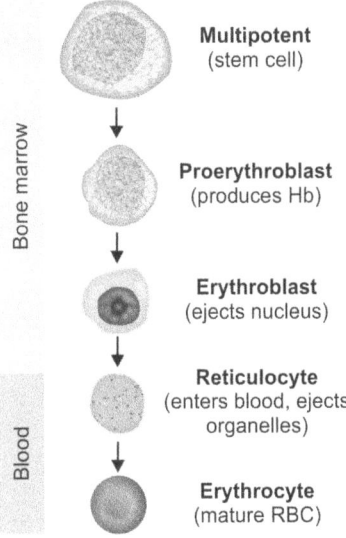

Fig. 4.5: Matuaration of RBCs.

two beta chains, each with a ring-like heme group containing an iron atom. Oxygen binds reversibly to these iron atoms and is transported through blood. Hemoglobin is responsible for the red color of the blood. Its structure consists of four subunits, typically a tetramer of alpha 2 beta 2, each containing a heme moiety in the ferrous state with iron. There are 141 amino acid residues in each alpha chain, and in each beta chains there are 146 residues. A normal adult male contains 14–16 g of hemoglobin per hundred mL of blood and a normal female contains 12–16 g per hundred mL of blood (**Fig. 4.6**).

The functions of hemoglobin are:
- Transport of Oxygen and Carbon dioxide in the body.
- Maintenance of acid-base balance
- Source of formation of Bilirubin

Hemolysis

The lifespan of RBC is about 120 days and their breakdown is carried out by phagocytic reticuloendothelial cells. This process is called **hemolysis**. Spleen, liver, and bone marrow are the major sites for hemolysis.

White Blood Cells or Leukocytes

White blood cells (WBCs), also called leukocytes, are the cells which actively participate in the immune system. They are involved in protecting the body against both infectious disease and foreign invaders. There are about 6,000–10,000 (every 8,000) WBCs per cubic millimeter in blood of an adult. The cytoplasm of WBCs contains nuclei and some have granules in their cytoplasm.

Classification of WBCs

They are classified into:
1. Granulocytes or polymorphonuclear leukocytes are classified as follow:
   a. *Neutrophils (polymorphs):* **Normal range: 2,500–6,000 per cubic mm.** They form the largest percentage of WBC approximately 42–60% of

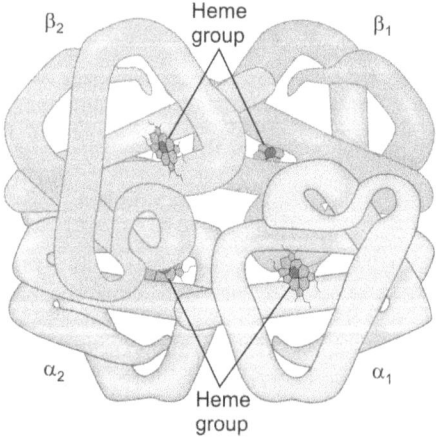

Fig. 4.6: Structure of hemoglobin.

the total WBCs. Neutrophils play a major role in the mechanism of defense. Their diameter varies from 10 to 12 µm in size. In their nucleus, there are 2-5 lobes that stain violet purple. Light pink stains in the cytoplasm with pinkish granules. In acute bacterial infections, the number increases **(Fig. 4.7)**.

b. *Eosinophils (Acidophils):* **Normal range: 40–400/µL.** These cells are slightly larger than neutrophils (12–14 µm). There are several wide, round/oval orange-pink granules in the cytoplasm of eosinophils. Allergic reactions such as asthma, food, and drug sensitivities are growing. The normal number of eosinophils is 2–4% of the total WBCs **(Fig. 4.8)**.

c. *Basophils:* The basophils are the rarest of the white blood cells. They are difficult to find in human blood because they constitute only 0.5–1% of total number of leukocytes. The nucleus is kidney-shaped or lobulated. They excrete two chemicals that aid in the body's defenses—histamine and heparin **(Fig. 4.9)**.

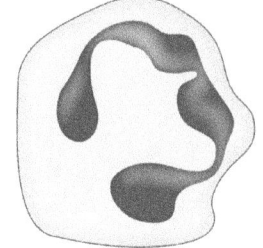

Fig. 4.7: Image of neutrophil.

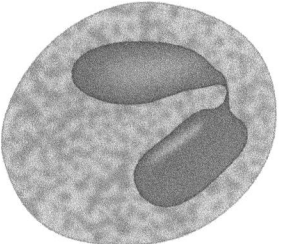

Fig. 4.8: Image of eosinophil.

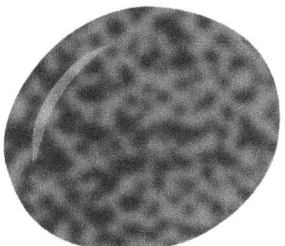

Fig. 4.9: Image of basophil.

2. **Agranular leukocytes:** They are divided into the following:
   a. *Lymphocytes:* It measures about 15–20 microns. They are associated with the body's defense mechanism. Lymphocytes are characterized by having a deeply stained nucleus and a comparatively small amount of cytoplasm. They are around 20–25%. Lymphocytosis is seen in viral infections, particularly in children **(Fig. 4.10)**.
   They are of two types:
   i. Small lymphocyte: Equal in size to mature erythrocyte or smaller, around nucleus filing the cells, can be pale blue cytoplasm containing Azure granules.
   ii. Large lymphocyte: It measures 10–40 microns, nuclear is large and around, cytoplasm containing azure granules.
   b. *Monocytes:* **Normal range: 700–1500/µL.** Monocytes range from 14 to 18 µm in diameter and are the largest WBCs. They have a centrally

Fig. 4.10: Image of lymphocytes.

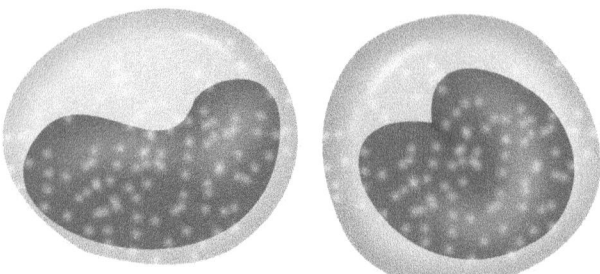

Fig. 4.11: Image of monocytes.

located nucleus that stains pale violet. They are around 3–8% wide and "horseshoe" shaped. Their cytoplasm stains are light greyish blue and contain dust-like granules of reddish blue and a few clear vacuoles. They circulate in the blood and are strongly phagocytic and motile. Monocytosis is seen in bacterial infections (e.g., tuberculosis) and protozoan infections (**Fig. 4.11**).

Platelets or Thrombocytes

They are small non-nucleated disc-shaped cells derived from megakaryocyte in red bone marrow. Platelets, also called thrombocytes (**thromb + cyte, "blood clot cell"**), are a component of blood whose function is to stop bleeding by clumping and clotting blood vessel injuries.
Normal range: 150,000–400,000/µL.

BLOOD GROUP

The blood group was found by Karl Landsteiner. The blood group system of ABO is used to categorize human beings' blood.

There are glycoproteins on the surface of the red cell and glycolipids that function as antigen. They are called blood group antigens. These antigens are present as antigen.

It can be present on the surface or protrude from the red cell's membrane. An immune reaction may take place, if introduced into a person who lacks the antigen.

An individual who donates blood is a donor. A recipient is a person who collects blood. If the donation of blood does not match that of the recipient, after transfusion, the incompatibility results in agglutination and lysis of donated red blood cells. This can lead to extreme disease and can cause death.

The antigens and a corresponding antibody in each blood group are shown in **Table 4.1**.

Rhesus System

The Rhesus factor is present on RBCs membranes. Individuals who have rhesus on their RBC are rhesus-positive (Rh +ve) and those who lack Rh antigen are designated as rhesus negative (Rh –ve). If a Rh-positive blood is given to

Chapter 4: Introduction to Cardiovascular System: Blood

TABLE 4.1: Antigens and corresponding antibodies.

Group	Antigen	Antibody
A	A	B
B	B	A
AB	AB	None
O	None	Anti A, Anti B

a Rh-negative person, no immediate reaction occurs. But during a second transfusion, the Rh negative person develops Anti-Rh agglutinin, which leads to agglutination of the reaction.

Erythroblastosis Fetalis

In this condition the fetus of Rh-negative mother and Rh-positive father is Rh positive. This may lead to serious complications as Rh antigen will travel from the fetus to Mother's blood. When these antibodies reach the fetus, they produce severe hemolytic reactions, which may lead to death of the fetus.

Clotting of Blood (Coagulation of Blood)

When a blood vessel is damaged bleeding occurs. Loss of blood is stopped by a formation of blood clot. Blood clotting is a defense mechanism of the body and prevents loss of blood from the site of injury. The formation of blood clot depends upon 12 factors.

Nomenclature for blood coagulation factors:
- **Factor I:** Fibrinogen
- **Factor II:** Prothrombin
- **Factor III:** Thromboplastin
- **Factor IV:** Calcium
- **Factor V:** Labile factor
- **Factor VI:** Unassigned
- **Factor VII:** Stable factor
- **Factor VIII:** Antihemophilic factor
- **Factor IX:** Christmas factor
- Factor V and VII are required for conversion of damaged tissue into thromboplastin. Factor VIII is an antihemophilic factor. Absence of Factor VIII leads to disease called hemophilia.

DISORDERS OF BLOOD

Anemia

Anemia is a state of decreased red cell mass of blood leading to decreased oxygen carrying capacity of the body. Red cell indices are useful in classifying anemia.

Chapter 4: Introduction to Cardiovascular System: Blood

TABLE 4.2: Classification of anemia.

Category	Anemia
Microcytic	Iron deficiency anemia, sideroblastic anemia, thalassemia
Macrocytic	Aplastic anemia vitamin B_{12} deficiency anemia
Normocytic	Hemolytic anemia and bone marrow suppression

Clinical features of anemia: There is usually shortness of breath (particularly on exercise), weakness, lethargy, palpitation, and headaches. In older subjects, symptoms of cardiac failure, angina pectoris, or intermittent claudication or confusion may be present.

Anemia can also be classified based on the size of the red blood cells and amount of hemoglobin in each cell **(Table 4.2)**.

Iron Deficiency Anemia

Incidence: This is the most prevalent type of anemia found globally and in India. It is seen in all age groups, but it is more common in age-bearing females and in infants.

Cause: Iron is one of the most common elements in the crust of the earth, yet iron shortages are the most common cause of anemia. This is because the body has a restricted capacity to absorb iron and excess iron loss is regular due to bleeding. It is caused by iron deficiency, which is necessary for normal hemoglobin production.

Megaloblastic Anemia

These are a group of disorders with abnormally large red cells due to faulty DNA synthesis and nuclear cytoplasmic asynchrony, resulting in anemia.

Cause: Vitamin B_{12}, or cobalamin and folic acid, are necessary for normal DNA synthesis. Megaloblastic anemia occurs due to one or both of these vitamins being deficient.

Pathogenesis: There is a deficiency in DNA synthesis in megaloblastic anemia, although RNA synthesis remains unimpaired. Due to hemoglobin being synthesized in excess during the delay, there is impaired cell division. As a consequence, erythroid precursors are formed as a result of this enlargement. All proliferating cells are affected by these changes.

Aplastic Anemia

Definition: Aplastic anemia is a condition in which red cells, white cells, and platelets are not produced by the bone marrow, resulting in PANCYTOPENIA.

Etiology: Bone marrow failure may be: (1) Congenital or inherited-called Fanconi anemia (2) Secondary to drugs, toxins, chemicals, exposure to radiation, or postspecific viral infections (3) Idiopathic, if the cause is unknown.

Clinical characteristics: The patient has symptoms of anemia (fatigue, breathlessness, pallor) because red cells are not produced by the marrow. Since normal WBC production is impaired, he/she may also have repeated and severe infections. Because of thrombocytopenia, the patient might also have bleeding symptoms.

Hemolytic Anemia
It is due to increased red blood cell destruction. It occurs because of mechanical injury to red blood cells or malarial infection due to hereditary disorders.

Polycythemia (Erythrocytosis)
There is an abnormal increase in the number of red blood cells in this condition. Changes include an increase in hemoglobin above 17.5 g/dL in adult males and 15.5 g/dL in females, usually with an associated increase in the number of red cells (**above 6.0 × 1012/L in males and 5.5 × 1012/L in females and hematocrit in females**).

Disorders of WBC
- Leukopenia is a condition in which WBCs are reduced below normal that is less than 4,000 per cubic mm of blood.
- **Agranulocytosis:** Acute condition there is a great reduction in number of polymorphonuclear leukocytes.
- **Leukopenia:** Decrease in the number of white blood cells in the blood.
- **Leukocytosis:** Abnormal circulating leukocytes pathological conditions.
- **Leukemia:** It is a cancerous condition characterized by an overproduction of white blood cells.

Disorders of Platelets
Thrombocytopenia: Decrease in the number of platelet count, which results in petechial hemorrhage, increase in bleeding time, and defect in retraction of clot.

Disorders of Clotting
Hemophilia: This condition occurs due to the absence of factor VIII (and antihemophilic factor)
Thrombosis: International clotting of blood is called thrombosis. It may occur due to roughening and blood vessels, which may lead to deep vein thrombosis.

SUMMARY
- Blood is a specialized form of connective tissue, which circulates in a closed system of blood vessels and is composed of transparent fluid plasma in which different types of cells are suspended.
- Blood is alkaline in nature pH of 7.4 (normal ranges 7.35–7.5).
- Blood contains plasma (straw-colored fluid) and cells.

Contd...

Chapter 4: Introduction to Cardiovascular System: Blood

Contd...

- Plasma constitute:
  - Water: 91%
  - Dissolved substances
    - Protein: 8%
    - Salts: 0.9%
- Cellular content (formed elements) of blood:
  - Leukocyte or white blood cells
  - Erythrocytes or red blood cells
  - Thrombocytes or platelets
- **Functions of blood are:** (1) Respiration: Transporting oxygen from lungs to tissues and carbon dioxide from tissues to lungs, (2) Coagulation of blood, (3) Excretion: transport of metabolic wastes to the lungs, kidneys, intestine, and skin for removal, (4) Nutrition, (5) Transport hormones, (6) Maintain a normal acid-base balance of the body, (7) Regulation of water balance, (8) Regulation of body temperature, (9) Transport of metabolites, (10) Defense against infection.
- **Erythropoiesis:** The process of development of RBCs is called erythropoiesis.
- **Hemoglobin:** It is a conjugated protein that serves as a vehicle for transportation of oxygen and carbon dioxide.
- **The functions of hemoglobin are:** (1) Transport of oxygen and carbon dioxide in the body, (2) Maintenance of acid-base balance, (3) Source of formation of bilirubin.
- **Classification of WBCs:** (1) Granulocytes or polymorphonuclear leukocytes—again classified as follows: Neutrophils (polymorphs), Eosinophils (acidophils) and Basophils, (2) Agranular leukocytes—they are divided into the following: Lymphocytes and Monocytes.
- **Platelets or thrombocytes:** They are small non-nucleated disc-shaped cells derived from megakaryocyte in red bone marrow, are a component of blood whose function is to stop bleeding by clumping and clotting blood vessel injuries.
- **Blood group:** The antigens and a corresponding antibody in each blood group are as follows:

Group	Antigen	Antibody
A	A	B
B	B	A
AB	AB	None
O	None	Anti-A, Anti-B

- **Anemia:** Anemia is a state of decreased red cell mass of blood leading to decreased oxygen carrying capacity of body. Red cell indices are useful in classifying anemia.
- **Clotting of blood (coagulation of blood):** Blood clotting is a defense mechanism of the body and prevents loss of blood from the site of injury. The formation of blood clot depends upon 12 factors. Nomenclature for blood coagulation factors is described as:
  - Factor I: Fibrinogen
  - Factor II: Prothrombin
  - Factor III: Thromboplastin
  - Factor IV: Calcium

Contd...

Chapter 4: Introduction to Cardiovascular System: Blood

Contd...

- ➢ Factor V: Labile factor
- ➢ Factor VI: Unassigned
- ➢ Factor VII: Stable factor
- ➢ Factor VIII: Antihemophilic factor
- ➢ Factor IX: Christmas factor
- ➢ Factor V and VII are required for conversion of damaged tissue into thromboplastin.
- ➢ Factor VIII is an antihemophilic factor. Absence of Factor VIII leads to disease called hemophilia.
- Leukopenia is a condition in which WBCs are reduced below normal that is less than 4,000 per cubic mm of blood.
- **Agranulocytosis:** Acute condition, there is a great reduction in number of polymorphonuclear leukocytes.
- **Leukocytosis:** Abnormal circulating leukocytes pathological conditions.
- **Leukemia:** It is a cancerous condition characterized by an overproduction of white blood cells.
- **Thrombocytopenia:** Decrease in the number of platelet count, which results in petechial hemorrhage, increase in bleeding time, and defect in retraction of clot.
- **Hemophilia:** This condition occurs due to the absence of factor VIII (and antihemophilic factor)
- **Thrombosis:** International clothing of blood is called thrombosis. It may occur due to roughening and blood vessels, which may lead to death.

GLOSSARY

1. **Agglutination:** The clumping of red blood cells on the surface of the cells as a result of antibodies bound to antigens.
2. **Antibodies:** These are the proteins that the body creates to recognize antigens and neutralize or kill them. Antibodies provide bodies with a significant protection against any foreign microorganism—causing disease.
3. **Antigens:** Molecules that provide blood or other tissue cells with a particular signature or identity. In addition to bacteria and viruses, antigens are present on the surface of blood and other tissue cells.
4. **Amino acids** are organic compounds that are protein building blocks. There are 20 amino acids of various kinds.
5. **Bacteria:** It is a simple single-sided microscopic organism lacking chlorophyll and a membrane around its nuclei. By mitosis, it reproduces. Many bacterial organisms are parasites of humans and other plants and animals.
6. **Enzymes:** It is a biological catalyst that speeds up chemical responses. The molecules upon which **enzymes** may act are called substrates, and the **enzyme** converts the substrates into different molecules known as products.
7. **Hormones:** Substances formed by specialized cells (usually proteins) that can move to other parts of the body where they influence chemical reactions and control different cellular functions. For example, with insulin.
8. **Albumin:** It is the liver's most abundant plasma protein. Different substances are transported by albumin, including bilirubin, fatty acids, metals, ions, and hormones.

Chapter 4: Introduction to Cardiovascular System: Blood

9. **Blood:** It is a liquid connective tissue made up of erythrocytes, leukocytes, and platelets and a plasma—called extracellular fluid matrix.
10. **Fibrinogen:** This is a plasma protein that is formed in the liver and is involved in blood coagulation.
11. **Lipids:** It is a water-insoluble macro biomolecule soluble in nonpolar solvents including fats, waxes, oils, hormones, etc.
12. **Plasma:** It is a liquid straw-colored medium in the blood that carries red cells, white cells, platelets, etc. Much of the volume of the blood consists of plasma.

LONG ANSWER TYPE QUESTIONS

1. Discuss in detail about the composition of blood and blood group system.
2. What is hemopoiesis? Discuss in detail disorders of blood.

SHORT ANSWER TYPE QUESTIONS

1. Give a brief account of RBCs.
2. What is blood coagulation.
3. What is plasma protein.

MULTIPLE CHOICE QUESTIONS

1. Which of the following statements about blood is true?
    a. Blood is about 20% water.
    b. Blood is slightly more acidic than water.
    c. Blood is slightly more viscous than water.
    d. Blood is slightly more salty than sea water.
2. Which of the following statements about albumin is true?
    a. It is the most abundant plasma protein.
    b. It is produced by specialized leukocytes called plasma cells.
    c. It draws water out of the blood vessels and into the body's tissues.
    d. None of the above
3. Which of the following plasma proteins is not produced by the liver?
    a. Fibrinogen
    b. Alpha globulin
    c. Immunoglobulin
    d. Beta globulin
4. What is the average life-span of RBCs?
    a. 8–10 days
    b. 120 days
    c. 1 years
    d. 3 years
5. What is the main function of neutrophil?
    a. Liberate heparin
    b. It has opposite effect to histamine
    c. Destroys bacteria with lymphocytes
    d. Blood clotting

ANSWERS KEY

1. c   2. a   3. c   4. b   5. c

Chapter 4: Introduction to Cardiovascular System: Blood

ATLAS
Identify and label the diagrams.

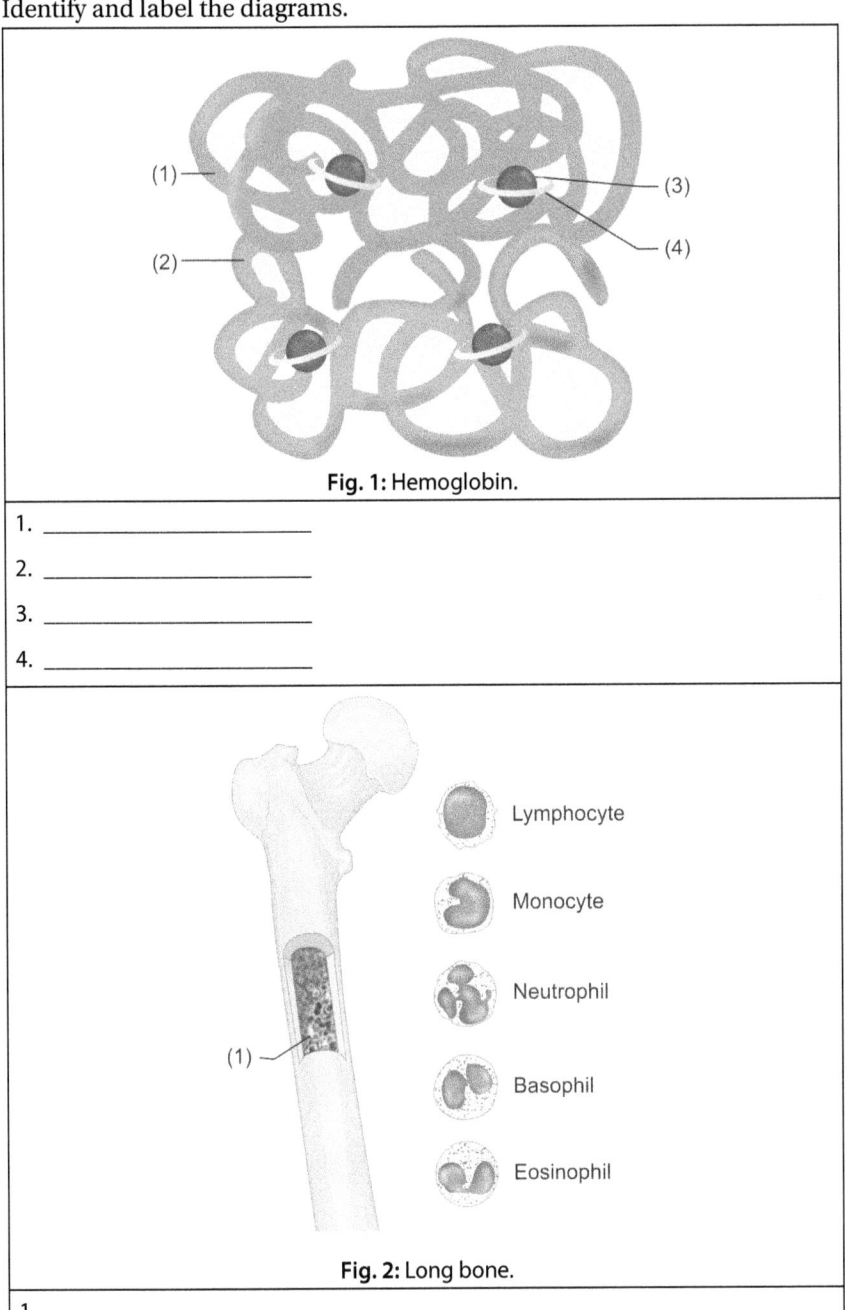

Fig. 1: Hemoglobin.

1. _____
2. _____
3. _____
4. _____

Fig. 2: Long bone.

1. _____

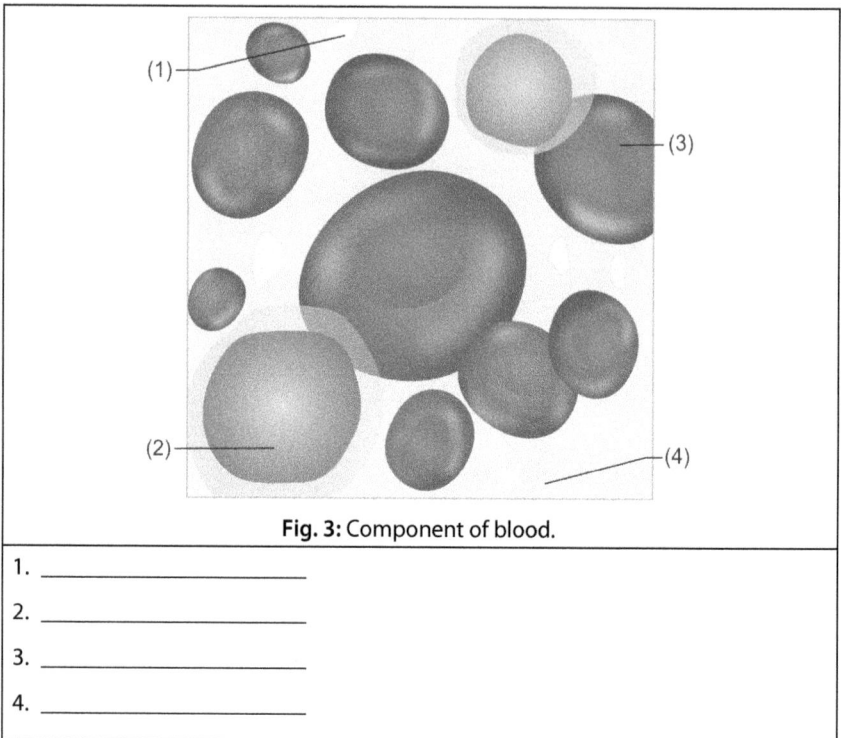

Fig. 3: Component of blood.

1. _____
2. _____
3. _____
4. _____

CHAPTER 5

Cardiovascular System: Heart

INTRODUCTION

Cardiovascular system is one of the most important systems of our body. The survival of the cells in our body depends on the availability of food, oxygen, and gases.

These functions are carried out by the cardiovascular system. The cardiovascular system consists of **heart, blood, and blood vessels**. Blood is a medium through which different materials are transported.

Common Terms

Blood Vessels

Blood vessels are very small tubes of different diameters. They can be as tiny as 0.5 mm or 3 cm in diameter at most. If the average adult had all the blood vessels and spread them out in one line, the line would be 100,000 miles long. Blood vessels such as lungs, arterioles, nerves, venules, and capillaries are of various kinds.

Arteries and Arterioles

Arteries and arterioles are the blood vessels that bring blood to a separate part of the body from the heart. Clean blood (oxygenated blood) is carried away from the heart by the arteries.

Arterioles are small arterial branches that are subdivided into capillaries. Capillaries bind veins to the arteries.

The arteries deliver to the capillaries the oxygen-rich blood, where the capillaries then deliver the waste-rich blood to the veins to return to the lungs and heart for transport.

Veins and Venules

Veins bring blood from various parts of the body back to the heart. Some veins have valves that keep the blood from flowing back. (Arteries do not need valves because there is very strong pressure from the heart that enables blood flow in one direction only).

HEART

The heart is a conical muscular organ that is hollow and weighs between 200 and 250 gram. The heart's size is about the fist of one's hand (**Fig. 5.1**).

Chapter 5: Cardiovascular System: Heart

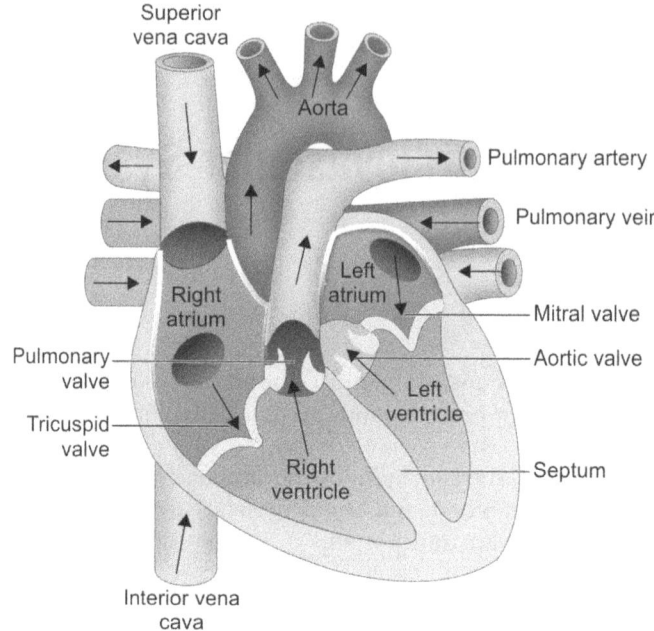

Fig. 5.1: Structure of heart.

Heart Position

Heart is situated between the lungs, in the thoracic cavity and behind the sternum, in the thorax (mediastinum). The heart's two-thirds section is inclined to the left side rather than the right side.

The apex of the heart can be felt approximately 5 cm to the left of the midline in the 5th intercostal, a little below the left nipple.

Heart Structure

Heart has three layers: Pericardium, myocardium, and endocardium.
1. **Pericardium:** The pericardium is called the outer lining. It comprises two layers of visceral pericardium and parietal pericardium, which are found between the two pericardial fluids. The fluid helps to decrease the pressure inside the pericardial sac as the heart moves.
2. **Myocardium:** The myocardium is known as the middle layer. It is a specialized fiber of the cardiac muscle found only in the heart.
3. **Endocardium:** The innermost layer of heart. It is a specialized cardiac muscle fiber found only in the heart.

Heart's Interior

The heart is separated by the interatrial and interventricular septum into the right portion of the left side. The heart consists of four chambers known as the: (1) right atrium, (2) left atrium, (3) right ventricle, and (4) left ventricle.

Chapter 5: Cardiovascular System: Heart

Heart's Valves

Dependent on the pressure in the chambers, the valves between the atrium and ventricles open and close. The tricuspid valves are situated in between the right ventricle and right atrium. The opening between left atrium and left ventricle is guarded by a bicuspid valve.

Blood Vessels Attached to the Heart

One of the major vessels is the heart, such as the superior vena cava, the inferior vena cava, the pulmonary artery, the pulmonary vein, and the aorta.

The cardiovascular system is a dual system, meaning that there are two distinct blood supply systems: Pulmonary and systemic circulation.

The human heart consists of two independent pumps, the right side (right atrium and ventricle) pumping the circulation of deoxygenated blood and the left side (left atrium and ventricle) pumping the circulation of oxygenated blood (**Fig. 5.2**).

Venae Cavae

Collectively, the superior and inferior vena cavae are called venae cavae. The venae cavae are involved in circulation alongside the aorta. These veins bring deoxygenated blood to the heart from the body, emptying it into the right side of the heart's atrium. The venae cavae are not isolated by valves from the right atrium.

Superior Vena Cava

Large and small veins bringing deoxygenated blood from the upper half of the body to the right atrium are the superior veins.

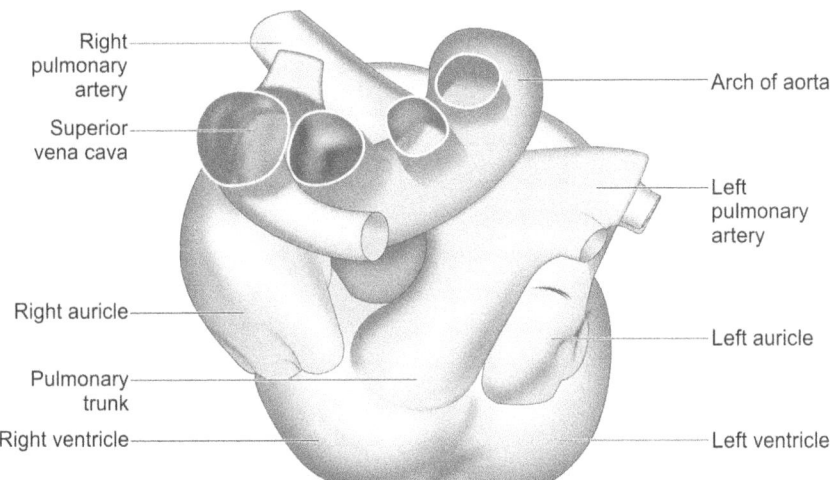

Fig. 5.2: Blood vessels attached to heart.

Inferior Vena Cava

Inferior vena cava is the biggest vein in the body and brings deoxygenated blood directly into the heart from the lower half of the body.

Aorta

In circulation, it is the largest of the arteries. From the left ventricle, blood is pumped into the aorta through the aortic valve. It is elastic in nature, which helps to regulate blood pressure.

Pulmonary Arteries

To absorb oxygen and unload carbon dioxide, the pulmonary arteries carry deoxygenated blood from the right ventricle into the alveolar capillaries of the lungs. Deoxygenated blood is carried away by these arteries, away from the heart.

Pulmonary Veins

The pulmonary veins transfer oxygenated blood from the lungs to the heart's left atrium. Both the pulmonary arteries and the veins are part of the lung circulation.

Conduction System of the Heart

There are specialized cells in the myocardium through which the impulses for cardiac contraction are transmitted in the heart (**Fig. 5.3**). The conduction system of the heart consists of:

- **Sinoatrial node (SA node):** It is known as a pacemaker. It initiates the contraction of the heart
- **Atrioventricular node (AV node):** The impulse of contraction generated from SA node stimulates the AV mode.

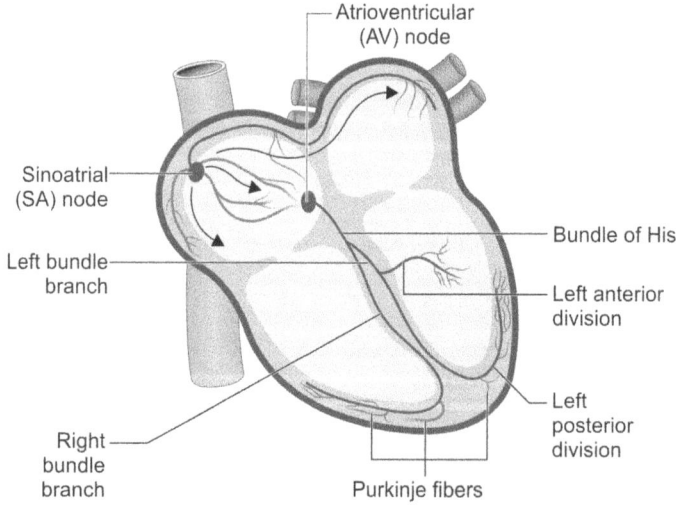

Fig. 5.3: Conduction system of heart.

Chapter 5: Cardiovascular System: Heart

- **Atrioventricular bundle (AV bundle or bundle of His):** From AV nodes impulses pass to bundle of his. The bundle of his passes through the interventricular septum, which divides into Purkinje fibers. The Purkinje fibers carry impulses of contraction from AV node to the ventricles causing them to contract. This contraction results in pumping of the blood into the aorta and pulmonary artery. Following this contraction the ventricles begin to relax and after complete relaxation another action potential starts SA node and next cycle starts.

Cardiac Cycle

The series of continuous contraction and relaxation of the heart is known as cardiac cycle. The beginning of one heartbeat to the beginning of next heartbeat is cardiac cycle. The average cardiac cycle of an adult is 72 cycles per minute.

It consists of two periods: Systole and diastole.

It includes:
- **Atrial systole:** It is a contraction of atria
- **Ventricular systole:** It is the contraction of the ventricle.
- **Cardiac diastole:** It is the relaxation of atria and ventricles.
- The length of each cardiac cycle is about 0.8 seconds

Cardiac Output

Cardiac output is defined as the volume of blood pumped out of the left ventricle or right ventricle into the aorta in 1 minute.

It can be measured by multiplying the stroke-volume (amount of blood ejected out per beat) into the heart rate.

For example, if the stroke volume is 70 mL and heart rate is 72 per minute, then cardiac output is as follows:

$$SV \times HR = CO$$
$$= 70 \text{ mL/beat} \times 72 \text{ beat/min}$$
$$= 5040 \text{ mL}.$$

In every minute around 5 L of blood is pumped by the heart. During vigorous exercise, it can increase up to 20 L per minute.

Heart Sounds

Two heart sounds can be heard separated by a pause. The first sound is lub (S1), which is due to the closure of atrioventricular valves. The second sound is dub (S2), which is due to the closure of aortic and pulmonary semilunar valves.

Third (S3) and fourth sounds (S4) are not heard normally.

Blood Pressure

Blood pressure is defined as the pressure exerted by blood on blood vessels. It is expressed as BP = 120/80 mm of Hg. Sphygmomanometer is used to measure blood pressure.

It is maintained by:
- Cardiac output
- Blood volume
- Elasticity of the arterial wall

Systolic blood pressure: Pressure exerted on the arteries during systole of the heart. It ranges from 100 to 120 mm Hg

Diastolic blood pressure: Pressure exerted on the arteries during diastole of the heart. It ranges from 60 to 80 mm Hg.

Electrocardiogram (ECG)

Electrocardiogram is a simple test, which is used to study heart's rhythm and electrical activity. The electrodes are placed on the skin and electrical activity is noted, any deviation from normal ECG may suggest cardiac abnormality.

Normally, 12 leads ECG is usually taken while lying down position. In a conventional 12 leads are placed in limbs and on the surface of chest. It takes around 10 seconds to record an ECG **(Fig. 5.4)**.

There are three main components of ECG.
1. **P-wave:** Represents the depolarization of the atria.
2. **QRS complex:** Represents the depolarization of the ventricles.
3. **T-wave:** Represents the repolarization of the ventricles.

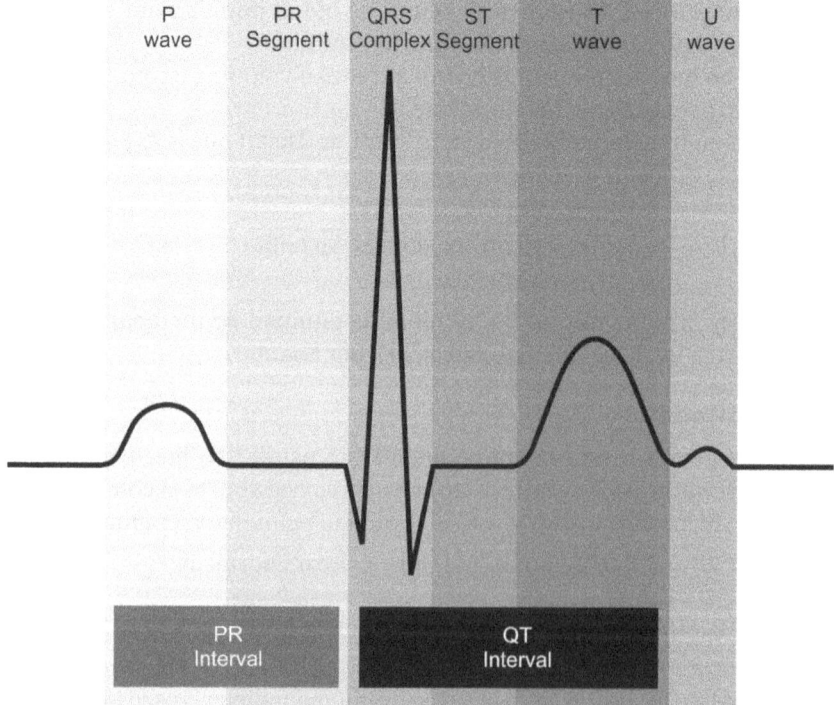

Fig. 5.4: Components of ECG.

Chapter 5: Cardiovascular System: Heart

ECG Leads (12 Leads)
Lead I, II, III, aVF, aVL, aVR, V_1, V_2, V_3, V_4, V_5, and V_6 (**Table 5.1**).

TABLE 5.1: ECG leads.

Category	Leads
Inferior leads	II, III, aVF
Lateral leads	I, aVL, V_5, and V_6 (aVF)
Septal leads	V_1 and V_2
Anterior leads	V_3 and V_4

SUMMARY

- **Blood vessels:** Blood vessels are very small tubes of different diameters. They can be as small as 0.5 mm in diameter or as largest 3 cm in diameter.
- **Arteries and arterioles:** These are the blood vessels, which carry blood away from the heart to a different parts of the body.
- **Veins and venules:** Veins carry the blood back to the heart from different parts of the body.
- The heart is a hollow, conical, muscular organ, which weighs about 200–250 gram. The size of the heart is about one's own hand fist.
- **Position of heart:** It is located in the thorax (mediastinum) between the lungs. In the thoracic cavity and behind the sternum.
- Heart has three layers, namely pericardium, myocardium, and endocardium.
- The heart is made up of four chambers known as: (1) right atrium, (2) left atrium, (3) right ventricle, and (4) left ventricle.
- The tricuspid valves are situated in between the right ventricle and right atrium. The opening between left atrium and left ventricle is guarded by a bicuspid valve.
- **The venae cavae:** These veins carry deoxygenated blood from the body into the heart, emptying it into the atrium of the right side of the heart.
- **Superior vena cava:** It carries deoxygenated blood from the upper half portion the body to the right atrium.
- **Inferior vena cava:** It carries deoxygenated blood from the lower half the body directly into the heart.
- **Aorta:** It is elastic in nature that helps in maintaining the pressure of blood.
- **Pulmonary arteries:** The pulmonary arteries carry deoxygenated blood from the right ventricle into the alveolar capillaries of the lungs to take up oxygen and unload carbon dioxide.
- **Pulmonary veins:** It carries oxygenated blood from the lungs to the left atrium of the heart.
- **Sinoatrial node (SA node):** It is known as a pacemaker. It initiates the contraction of the heart.
- **Atrioventricular node (AV node):** The impulse of contraction generated from SA node stimulates the AV node.
- **Atrioventricular bundle (AV bundle or bundle of His):** From AV nodes impulses pass to bundle of His.
- The average cardiac cycle of an adult is 72 cycles per minute.
- **Cardiac output:** It is defined as the volume of blood pumped out of the left ventricle or right ventricle into the aorta in one minute.
- **Blood pressure:** It is defined as the pressure exerted by blood on blood vessels.

Chapter 5: Cardiovascular System: Heart

GLOSSARY

1. **Heart:** A fist-sized muscular organ in the chest that pumps blood.
2. **Ventricle:** One of two lower chambers of the heart that receives blood and pumps it out into pulmonary or systemic circulation.
3. **Myocardium:** The middle of the three layers forming the wall of the heart.
4. **Pericardium**—a serous membrane that surrounds and protects the heart.
5. **Endocardium:** A thin serous membrane that lines the interior of the heart and valves.
6. **Pulmonary arteries:** The arteries that take deoxygenated blood away from the right side of the heart and into the capillaries of the lungs for the purpose of gas exchange.
7. **Aorta:** The great artery, which carries the blood from the heart into systemic circulation.
8. **Venae cavae:** The two large vessels, the superior and inferior vena cava, that bring deoxygenated blood from systemic circulation to the heart.

LONG ANSWER TYPE QUESTIONS

1. Draw a neat and labeled diagram of heart? Name the three layers of the heart and explain their functions.
2. Discuss in detail conduction system of heart.

SHORT ANSWER TYPE QUESTIONS

Write short note on:
1. Cardiac cycle.
2. Cardiac output.
3. Blood pressure.

MULTIPLE CHOICE QUESTIONS

1. From where heartbeat starts:
   a. Right ventricle
   b. Right atrium
   c. Left atrium
   d. Left ventricle
2. Valves are found in:
   a. Capillaries
   b. Arteries
   c. Arterioles
   d. Veins
3. What is the instrument for measuring blood pressure called?
   a. Electrocardiogram
   b. Anemometer
   c. Stethoscope
   d. Sphygmomanometer
4. Which of the following veins does not carry deoxygenated blood?
   a. Hepatic vein
   b. Pulmonary vein
   c. Renal vein
   d. Hepatic portal vein
5. Where does impulse initiate from:
   a. SA node
   b. AV node
   c. Vagus nerve
   d. Cardiac nerve

ANSWERS KEY

1. b   2. d   3. d   4. b   5. a

Chapter 5: Cardiovascular System: Heart

ATLAS

Identify and label the diagrams.

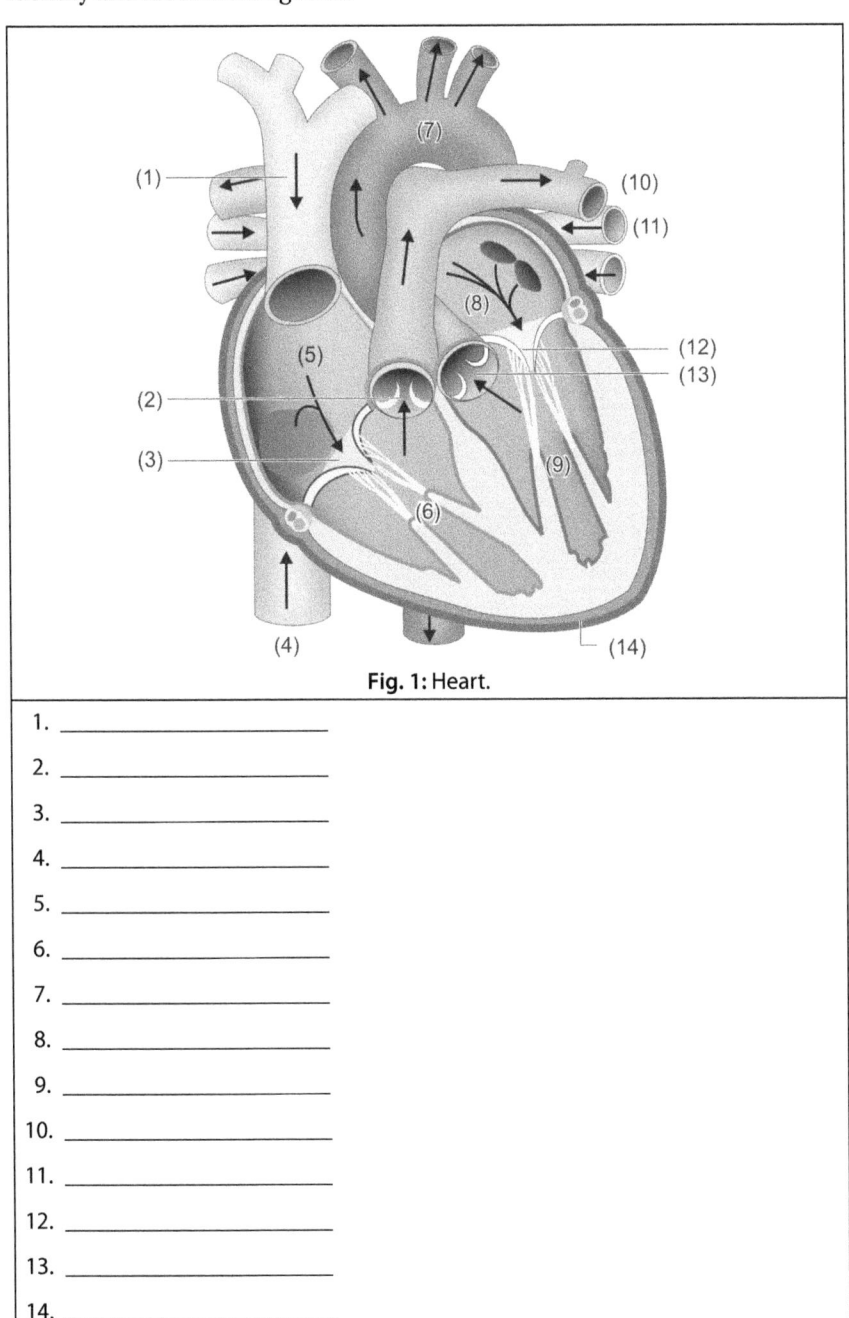

Fig. 1: Heart.

1. _____
2. _____
3. _____
4. _____
5. _____
6. _____
7. _____
8. _____
9. _____
10. _____
11. _____
12. _____
13. _____
14. _____

Chapter 5: Cardiovascular System: Heart

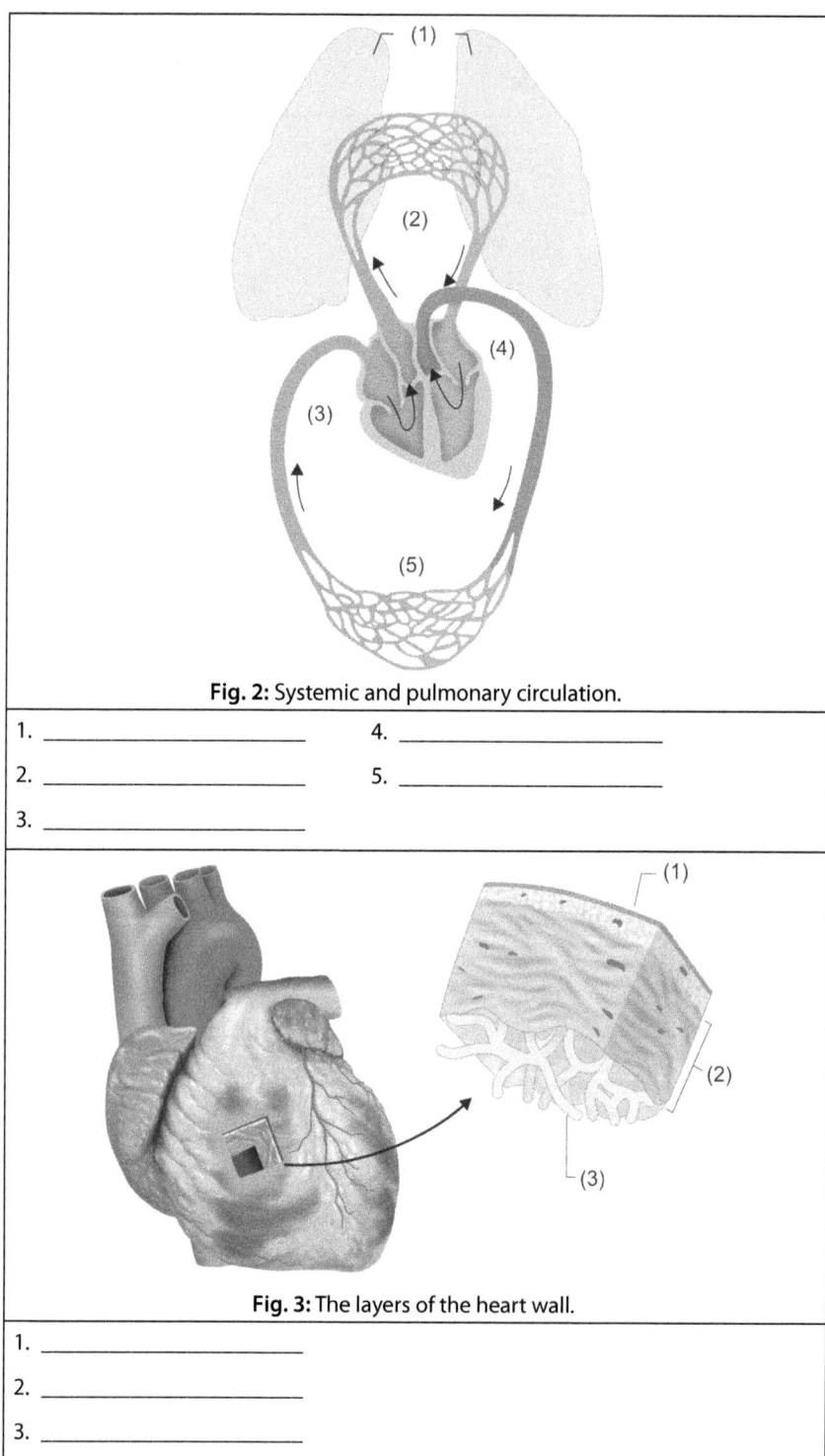

Fig. 2: Systemic and pulmonary circulation.

1. _____
2. _____
3. _____
4. _____
5. _____

Fig. 3: The layers of the heart wall.

1. _____
2. _____
3. _____

Chapter 5: Cardiovascular System: Heart

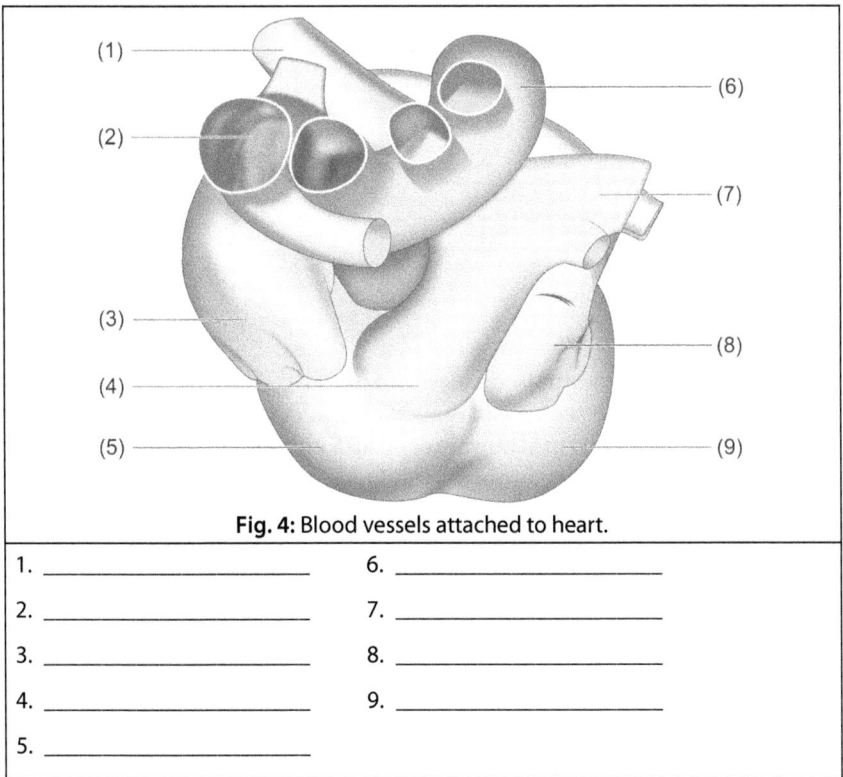

Fig. 4: Blood vessels attached to heart.

1. _____
2. _____
3. _____
4. _____
5. _____
6. _____
7. _____
8. _____
9. _____

CHAPTER 6

Respiratory System

INTRODUCTION

Respiratory system is structurally divided into upper and lower respiratory system. **Upper respiratory system** consists of nose, nasal cavity, pharynx (throat), and larynx portion above vocal cord. **Lower respiratory system** involves larynx portion below the vocal cord, trachea, bronchi, and lung.

Functionally, respiratory system has two divisions, one is respiratory zone, other one is conducting zone. **Respiratory zone** consists of tubes and tissues such as bronchioles, alveoli, alveolar sac, and duct. This is the main site for gaseous exchange. **Conducting zone** contains the connecting tube and cavities inside or outside the lungs such as nasal cavity, nose, larynx, pharynx, trachea, bronchi, and bronchioles. Their main function is to warm, moisten, and filter the air and take it to the lungs. Let us discuss all structures one by one.

Nose

- Nose is divided into external and internal part.
- External part, which is visible on our face and supported by bone, hyaline cartilage, and covered with skin and muscles, lined with mucous membrane.
- Internal part of the nose is also known as nasal cavity. It is a spacious cavity, which is covered with the mucous membrane and muscles.
- Anteriorly, nasal cavity merges with external nose and posteriorly it continues with pharynx (**Fig. 6.1**).

Pharynx

- Pharynx is also known as throat.
- It is a funnel-shaped tube.
- It is about 13 cm long, it starts from internal nares and extends till inferior cartilage of larynx that is cricoid cartilage.
- The superior portion of the pharynx is nasopharynx; it lies posterior to the nasal cavity.
- The posterior wall of pharynx contains pharyngeal tonsils or adenoids.
- The middle portion of pharynx is oropharynx, which is posterior to the oral cavity.
- Oropharynx contains the palatine and lingual tonsils.
- The inferior portion of the pharynx is laryngopharynx that begins at the level of hyoid bone.

Chapter 6: Respiratory System

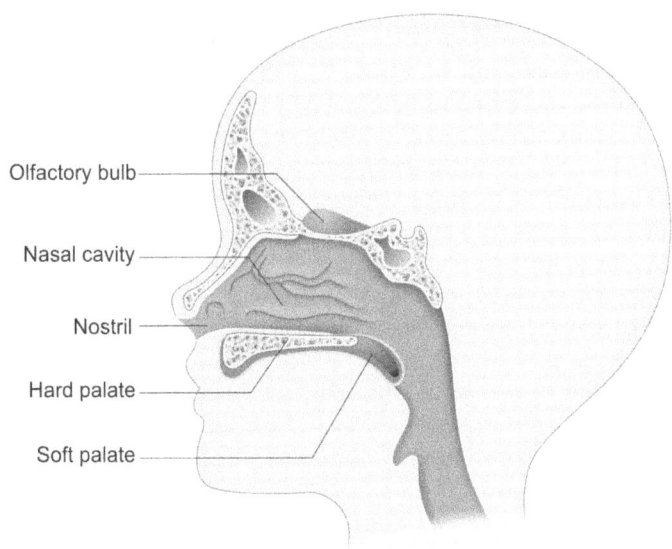

Fig. 6.1: Nose.

- Oropharynx and laryngopharynx serve both respiratory and digestive tracts, so they are lined with nonkeratinized stratified squamous epithelium (Fig. 6.2).

Disorders
- **Pharyngitis:** It is the inflammation of pharynx.
- **Tonsillitis:** It is inflammation of the tonsils due to infection.

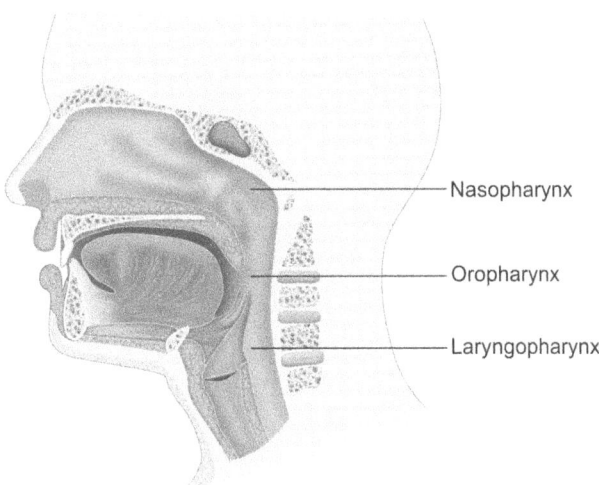

Fig. 6.2: Pharynx.

Larynx

- Larynx is also known as voice box.
- It connects laryngopharynx with trachea.
- Walls of larynx are made up of three single and three paired pieces of cartilage, therefore total nine pieces.
- Single cartilages are thyroid cartilage, epiglottis, and cricoid cartilage.
- Thyroid cartilage is also known as Adam's apple and gives the triangular shape to the anterior wall of larynx.
- Epiglottis, it is an elastic cartilage, which is a large and leaf-shaped piece.
- Cricoid cartilage, it forms the inferior wall of the larynx, and it is a ring of hyaline cartilage.
- Paired cartilages are arytenoid, which are triangular pieces cartilage, corniculate they are horn-shaped elastic cartilage, cuneiform cartilage (they are wedge-shaped that supports the epiglottis) **(Fig. 6.3)**.

Disorders

Laryngitis: Inflammation of the larynx.

Trachea

- It is also known as windpipe.
- It is about 12 cm long and 2.5 cm in diameter.
- It is situated anterior to the esophagus.
- Layers of trachea are mucosa, the deepest layer, submucosa, hyaline cartilage, and then superficial layer known as adventitia that is composed of areolar connective tissue.

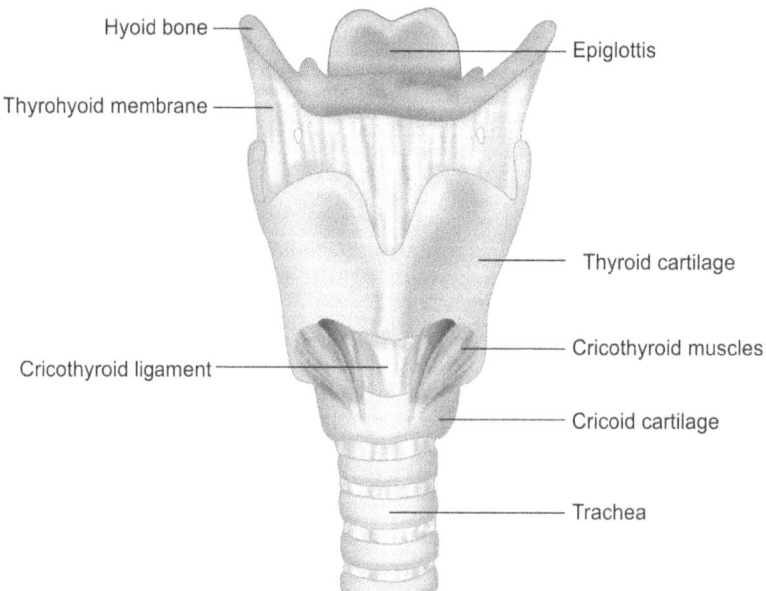

Fig. 6.3: Larynx.

Bronchi

- Trachea divides into right and left primary bronchus.
- Right primary bronchus goes into right lungs and left primary bronchus goes into left lungs.
- Right primary bronchus is shorter, wider, and vertical than left one.
- Primary bronchi line with pseudostratified ciliated columnar epithelium.
- Primary bronchi divide into secondary bronchi for each lobe of the lung.
- Right lung has three lobes, whereas the left has two lobes.
- Secondary bronchus is branched into tertiary and then into bronchioles.
- Bronchioles continue branching and the smaller branch is known as terminal bronchioles.
- Bronchial tree is the inverted tree that extends through the terminal bronchioles (**Fig. 6.4**).

Disorders

- **Bronchitis:** It is the inflammation of the bronchioles.
- **Bronchiectasis:** There is damage to the airways, which results in widening of the airways.
- **Bronchospasm:** It is the shrinkage of bronchioles.

Lungs

- It is a cone-shaped organ that lies in the thoracic cavity.
- Lungs are separated through the heart and by the help of mediastinum.
- Each lung is protected by the double-layered serous membrane called pleural membrane.
- There are two types of pleura parietal and visceral pleura. Parietal lines the superficial thoracic cavity whereas visceral covers the lungs.

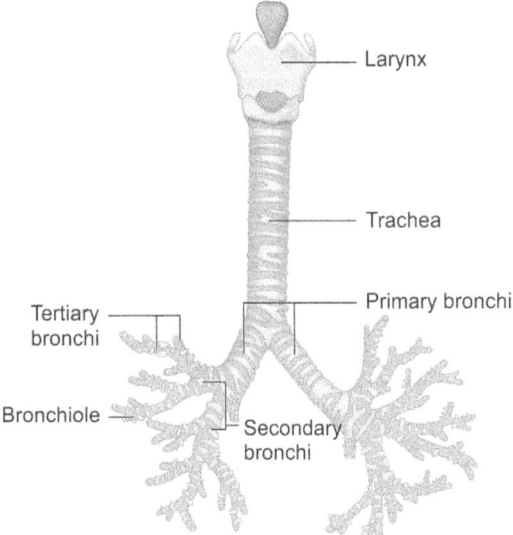

Fig. 6.4: Bronchi.

Chapter 6: Respiratory System

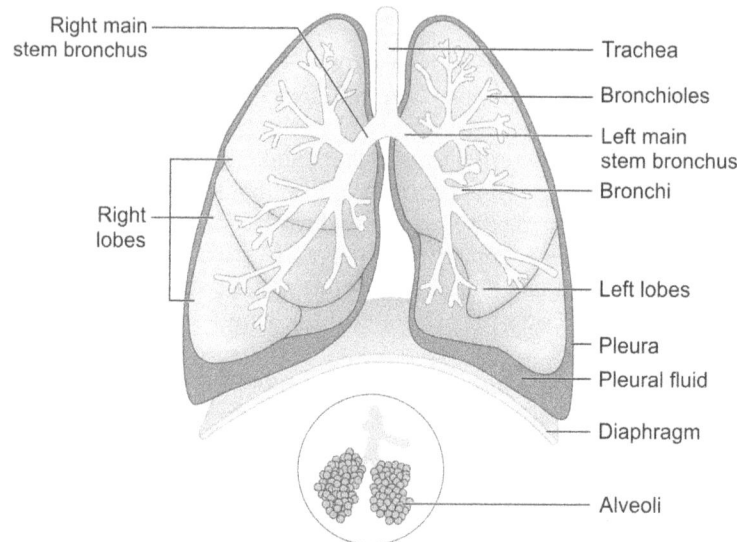

Fig. 6.5: Lungs.

- Pleural cavity is the space between the parietal and visceral pleura. Pleural fluid is present in pleural cavity.
- The broad inferior portion of the lung is base, and the superior narrow portion is apex.
- The medial surface that is mediastinal contains a region named hilum via which all bronchi, nerves, pulmonary blood and lymphatic vessels enter and exit (Fig. 6.5).

Disorders
- **Asthma:** It is hypersensitivity of the airway in which person's airway becomes inflamed, narrow, and produces the extra mucus.
- **COPD:** It is the chronic obstructive pulmonary disease; it is a group of lung disease that causes the difficulty in breathing by causing airway blockage.
- **Pneumonia:** In this condition the air sacs are filled with fluid or pus.

Alveoli
- An alveolus is a cup-shaped structure that lines with simple squamous epithelium.
- An alveolar sac contains two or more alveoli.
- The wall of alveoli contains two types of cells, type I and type II alveolar cells.
- Type I are simple squamous cells that line the alveolar wall, their main function is gaseous exchange.
- Type II also called septal cells; these are cuboidal epithelium having microvilli present between type I cells. They secrete alveolar fluid and keep the air moist.
- Alveolar fluid contains the surfactant, which prevents alveoli from collapsing.

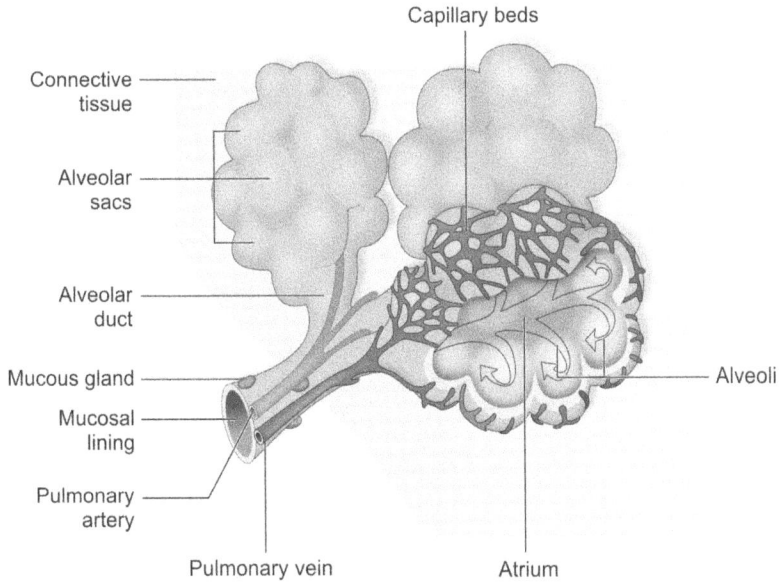

Fig. 6.6: Alveoli.

- Alveolar macrophages that remove dust particles and other dead cells from alveolar space **(Fig. 6.6)**.

FUNCTIONS OF RESPIRATORY SYSTEM

- Gaseous exchange: Exchange of oxygen and carbon dioxide.
- It aids in breathing.
- Larynx helps in production of sound.
- Nose helps in olfactory sensation (sensing the smell).
- Cilia in lungs help in protection from foreign particles and sweeps away dust.
- It also helps in acid-base balance.

PHYSIOLOGY OF RESPIRATION

Pulmonary Ventilation

The process of gaseous exchange is known as respiration. It involves pulmonary ventilation, external and internal respiration **(Fig. 6.7)**.
- **Pulmonary ventilation:** It is the inhalation and exhalation of air and exchange of air between the alveoli and the atmosphere.
- **External (pulmonary) respiration:** It is the exchange of gases between the alveoli and the pulmonary capillaries. In the pulmonary capillaries, blood gets the oxygen and loses carbon dioxide.
- **Internal (tissue) respiration:** It is the exchange of gases between the blood in systemic capillaries and tissue cells. In this the blood gets carbon dioxides and loses oxygen.

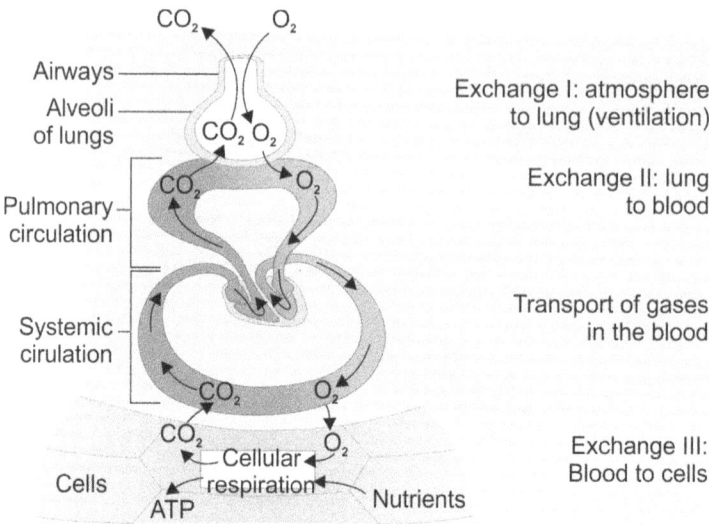

Fig. 6.7: Physiology of respiration.

Inhalation

- Breathing-in is known as inhalation.
- The inhalation involves the contraction of muscles such as diaphragm and external intercostals.
- Diaphragm is a dome-shaped skeletal muscle that covers the thoracic cavity.
- During inhalation the diaphragm contracts and descends downward.
- Another important muscle of inhalation is external intercostals, contraction of these muscles elevates the ribs, which helps in entering about 25% of air into the lungs.

Exhalation

- Breathing-out is known as exhalation.
- During exhalation there is no contraction involves. Therefore, exhalation is known as passive process.
- Exhalation results from elastic recoil of the chest wall and lungs and both of them have tendency to get back to normal shape after being stretched.
- Exhalation starts when inhalation muscles and diaphragm relax.

ALTERATIONS IN RESPIRATION

- **Apnea:** It is the cessation of breathing.
- **Dyspnea:** It is the difficulty in breathing.
- **Orthopnea:** It is the difficulty in breathing in upright position.
- **Wheezing:** It is the whistling sound during breathing.
- **Cheyne-Stokes respiration:** It is the abnormal pattern of breathing that is characterized by deeper and faster breathing followed by slowly decrease and then temporary episode of apnea.

Lung Volumes and Capacities
- **Tidal volume:** The volume of one breath is tidal volume. With each inhalation about 500 mL of air moves in and out of the lungs.
- **Minute volume:** Total volume of air inhaled and exhaled each minute is minute volume. It is calculated by respiratory rate multiplied by tidal volume.

    Minute volume = (Respiratory rate × Tidal volume)
    = 12 breath/min × 500 mL/breath
    = 6 L/min

- **Alveolar ventilation rate:** It is the volume of air per minute reaches the respiratory tract.
- **Inspiratory reserve volume:** By taking a deep breath, the additional deep breath taken in addition to normal one is known as inspiratory reserve volume.
- **Expiratory reserve volume:** When inhale normally but exhale forcefully results in exhalation of excessive air than normal, it is known as expiratory reverse volume.
- **Residual volume:** It is the amount of air that remains in the lungs after forceful expiration.
- **Inspiratory capacity:** It is the sum of tidal volume and inspiratory reserve volume.
- **Vital capacity:** It is the sum of inspiratory reserve volume, tidal volume, and expiratory reserve volume.
- **Total lung capacity:** It is the sum of vital capacity and residual volume.

EXCHANGE OF OXYGEN AND CARBON DIOXIDE
- **External respiration:**
  - It is also known as the pulmonary gas exchange.
  - It is the diffusion of air from the alveoli of lungs to the blood in pulmonary capillaries and the diffusion of carbon dioxide in opposite direction.
  - It converts the deoxygenated blood into oxygenated that comes from the right side of the heart. Then it returns to the left portion of the heart.
- **Internal respiration:**
  - It is also known as systemic gas exchange.
  - As soon as the oxygen leaves the blood stream, the oxygenated blood converted into the deoxygenated blood.
  - Internal respiration occurs in tissue throughout the body.

Control of Respiration
Respiratory center: Medulla oblongata and pons part of the brain is the respiratory center. Impulses send by them results in contraction of thorax and in the absence of impulses it relaxes. There are three respiratory centers medullary rhythmicity, pneumotaxic, and apneustic area.
1. **Medullary rhythmicity area:** The main function of this area to control the basic rhythm of respiration.

2. **Pneumotaxic area:** It is the regulatory area in pons of the brain. It helps in the coordination between the inhalation and exhalation.
3. **Apneustic area:** It is also present in the pons; it also helps in the coordination between the transition of inhalation and exhalation.

REGULATION OF THE RESPIRATORY CENTER

- **Cortical influences on respiration:** Cerebral cortex has connection with the respiratory center; therefore, we can voluntarily alter our breathing pattern, we can stop our breathing for a shorter period of time. It is useful as a protective factor as it can prevent the entry of water and irritating gases inside the lungs.
- **Chemoreceptor regulation of respiration:** Sensory neurons are responsible for the generation of chemoreceptors, which decide how deeply and quickly we can breathe:
  - Central chemoreceptors, which are present near the medulla oblongata they respond in the change of hydrogen ion concentration, pCO_2 or both in cerebrospinal fluid.
  - Peripheral chemoreceptors are present in the aorta; they are sensitive to the changes in hydrogen, pO_2 and pCO_2 in the blood.

SUMMARY

- Respiratory system is divided into upper and lower respiratory system.
- Nose can be described as external nose covered externally with skin and internal nasal cavity.
- Pharynx is also known as throat. There is nasopharynx, oropharynx, and laryngopharynx.
- Larynx is known as voice box; its wall is composed with the nine pieces of cartilages.
- Trachea is also known as windpipe, it is further dived into bronchi.
- Bronchi are divided into right and left primary bronchus that lead to the secondary then tertiary, terminal bronchioles and form the bronchial tree.
- Lungs have the pleural fluid-filled cavity known as pleural cavity.
- Respiration involves the pulmonary ventilation, external and internal respiration.
- Medulla oblongata and pons are the respiration control center in our brain.
- Cortical and chemoreceptors regulate the respiratory center.

GLOSSARY

1. **Internal nares:** It is the nostril.
2. **Adenoids:** They are the patch of tissue and part of lymphatic system, present behind the nose.
3. **Tonsils:** They are also the part of lymphatic system and are lump of tissues.
4. **Hyoid bone:** A U-shaped bone in the neck, it supports the tongue.
5. **Cartilage:** It is a smooth elastic tissue.
6. **Pons:** It is the part of the brainstem, helps in regulation of respiration.

Chapter 6: Respiratory System

7. **Medulla oblongata:** It is a stem-like structure. It is responsible for the involuntary functions.
8. **Mediastinum:** It is the division of thoracic cavity, it consists of the trachea along with esophagus, thymus gland, and heart.

LONG ANSWER TYPE QUESTIONS

1. Describe anatomical structure of lung along with labeled diagram.
2. Explain the physiology of respiration.
3. Define the following terms:
   a. Vital capacity
   b. Tidal volume
   c. Minute ventilation
   d. Larynx

MULTIPLE CHOICE QUESTIONS

1. Among these which is known as voice box?
   a. Pharynx
   b. Larynx
   c. Bronchi
   d. Trachea
2. Right lung is divided in how many lobes?
   a. 2
   b. 1
   c. 4
   d. 3
3. Respiratory system is made up of the lungs, trachea, and the:
   a. Esophagus
   b. Diaphragm
   c. Liver
   d. Gallbladder
4. The trachea is also known as:
   a. Windpipe
   b. Bronchus
   c. Bronchioles
   d. Lung
5. Tiny hair-like projections that sweep away dirt and mucus are known as:
   a. Cilia
   b. Flagella
   c. Macrophages
   d. Bronchioles

ANSWERS KEY

1. b   2. d   3. b   4. a   5. a

CHAPTER 7

Digestive System

INTRODUCTION

Nutrition is required for the healthy body that comes from the food, which we consume. Our body gets nutrition from the digested food. Digestion takes place in digestive system which comprises alimentary tract and accessory organs. Alimentary tract is also known as gastrointestinal tract or GI tract. The length of GI tract varies in a living person and cadaver. It is slightly long in cadaver due to loss of muscle tone. The length of GI tract in a living body is 7-9 meters and in cadaver its 9-12 meters. Alimentary canal consists of a mouth, pharynx, esophagus, stomach, small intestine, large intestine, rectum and anal canal. On the other hand (tongue, salivary glands, liver, Gallbladder, and pancreas) they are the pivotal accessory organs, which participate in the process of digestion.

In this chapter, we will have a detailed look at the digestive system in human beings, different organs of the digestive system and the mechanism of digestion in humans (**Fig. 7.1**).

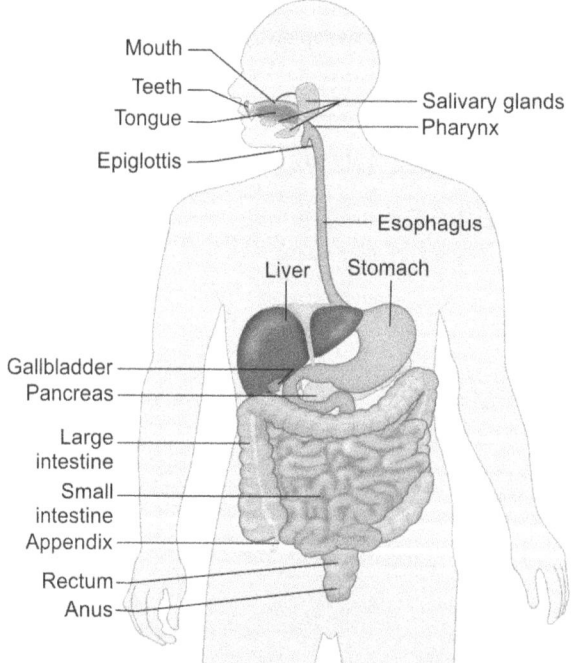

Fig. 7.1: Digestive system in human being.

BASIC PROCESSES OF DIGESTION

- **Ingestion:** Intake of food is known as ingestion.
- **Secretion:** After intake of food, there is gush of salivary secretions to moisten the food.
- **Mixing and propulsion:** Saliva mixes with the food to form the bolus and then the formed bolus propels downward that moves to esophagus.
- **Digestion:** It occurs in two phases; one is chemical digestion and other is mechanical digestion.
    - *Chemical digestion:* It is the release of secretions and enzymes for the breakdown and digestion of food. For example, saliva in mouth to mix and moisten the food, hydrochloric acid (HCl) in stomach to digest the food.
    - *Mechanical digestion:* It is the work done by the parts of digestive organ, like teeth to cut and grind the food, tongue helps in swallowing the food.
- **Absorption:** Maximum absorption occurs in small intestine via which the nutrients deliver to the body tissues and cells.
- **Defecation:** Our body does not absorb the whole food or nutrients that we eat. Some portion absorbed by our body and rest is converted into fecal or waste matter and then excrete out in the form of feces.

LAYERS OF GI TRACT

It is made up of four types of layers **(Fig. 7.2)**:
1. **Mucosa:** It is the inner-most layer of GI tract. Mucosa is made up of three layers that are nonkeratinized epithelium, lamina propria, which is made up of connective tissue and have blood and lymphatic vessels and muscularis mucosae that have thin layers of muscles.

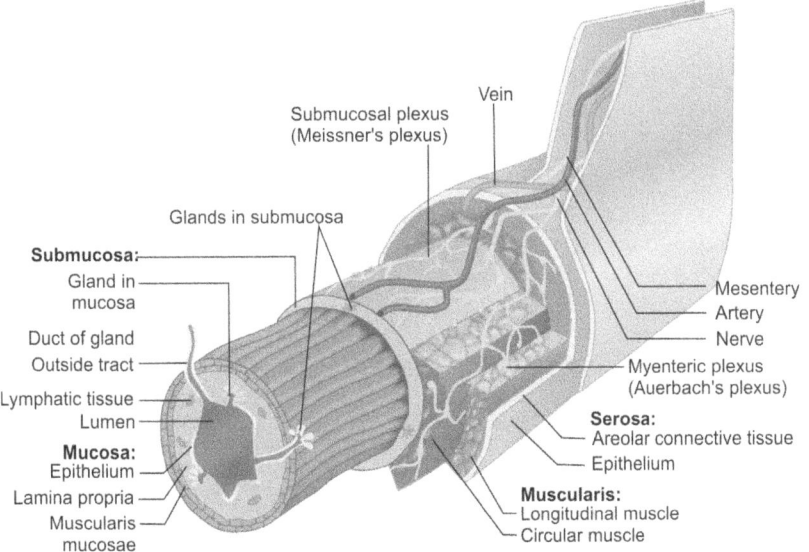

Fig. 7.2: Layers of GI tract.

2. **Submucosa:** Submucosa is also made up of connective tissue and comprises the blood and lymphatic vessels to carry the nutrients and reach it to the body parts. Submucosa consists of the submucosal plexus that is submucosal nerve network that aids in regulating the glandular secretions.
3. **Muscularis:** This layer is made up of skeletal and smooth muscles. Muscles in GI tract arranged in circular and longitudinal directions except in stomach where it is arranged obliquely also. Muscularis layer consists of the myenteric plexus that helps in muscular activity within GI tract such as peristalsis.
4. **Serosa/adventitia:** This is the outmost layer in the GI tract. They are made up of loose connective tissues, it has mucus to moisten the surface.

MOUTH

Mouth is also known as oral cavity, externally it is surrounded by skin that is known as cheeks and internally it is covered with nonkeratinized stratified epithelium which keep that area moisturized and wet. Other than this, mouth consists of a muscular tongue that bears taste buds, 16 pairs of teeth and salivary gland **(Fig. 7.3).**

- **Palate:** Mouth has a hard and a soft palate. Bony hard palate anteriorly present at the roof of the mouth and muscular soft palate present at posterior surface.
- **Uvula:** It is a hanging muscular fold that is covered with mucous membrane.
- **Vestibule:** It is the space between the lips, cheeks and teeth.

Association with Mouth
- **Anteriorly:** It is covered with lips.
- **Posteriorly:** It is in continuation with pharynx that is known as oropharynx

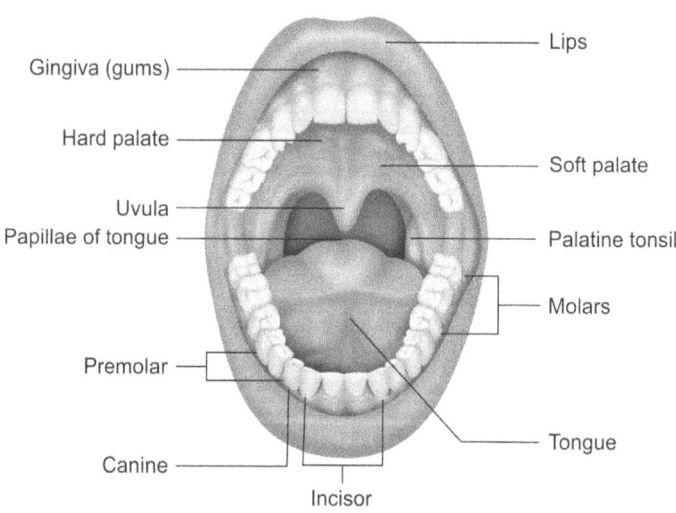

Fig. 7.3: Mouth (oral cavity).

- **Laterally:** It is surrounded with cheeks along with muscles of the cheek.
- **Superiorly:** Hard and soft palate present superiorly that is at the upper surface of the mouth.

Tongue
- It is a muscular organ.
- **Frenulum:** It is centrally divided portion that is made up of mucous membrane.
- One of the salivary glands is present under the tongue, known as sublingual gland.
- It consists of the papillae (nipple-like projections) that bear the taste buds but all papillae do not contain taste buds.

Types of Papillae
1. **Fungiform papillae:**
   - These are the mushroom-shaped papillae
   - They contain taste buds
2. **Circumvallate papillae:**
   - They are inverted v-shaped papillae.
   - Contains taste buds
3. **Foliate papillae:**
   - They are leaf-like papillae
   - Present at lateral surface of tongue and contains taste buds.
4. **Filiform papillae:**
   - Does not contain taste buds
   - They have sensory receptors **(Fig. 7.4)**.

Blood Supply
- **Venous drainage:** Lingual veins and internal jugular veins
- **Arterial supply:** Lingual artery, external carotid artery.

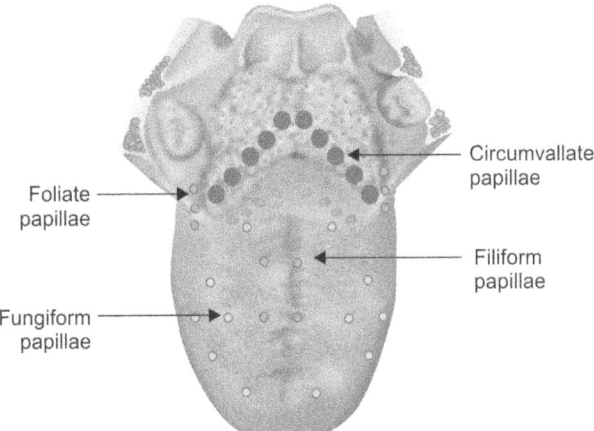

Fig. 7.4: Types of papillae.

Teeth

Dentition formula: 2123/2123
- **Incisors:** Central and lateral incisors (used for cutting)
- **Canine:** Use for tearing of food
- **Premolar:** 1st and 2nd premolar (used for crushing of food)
- **Molar:** 1st, 2nd, and 3rd molar (3rd molar also known as wisdom teeth), used for grinding.

Parts of Teeth
- **Enamel:** Hardest part of the teeth
- **Dentin:** It presents between enamel and cementum
- **Cementum:** It is a specialized bone-like substance that covers the root of the tooth.
- **Dental pulp:** It is the central part and filled with connective tissue (**Fig. 7.5**).

Blood Supply
- **Venous drainage:** Internal jugular veins
- **Arterial supply:** Maxillaries arteries

Salivary Glands

Salivary glands are the exocrine glands that secrete the saliva. There are three pairs of major salivary glands (**Fig. 7.6**). These are as follows:
1. **Parotid gland:** These are present near the ears.

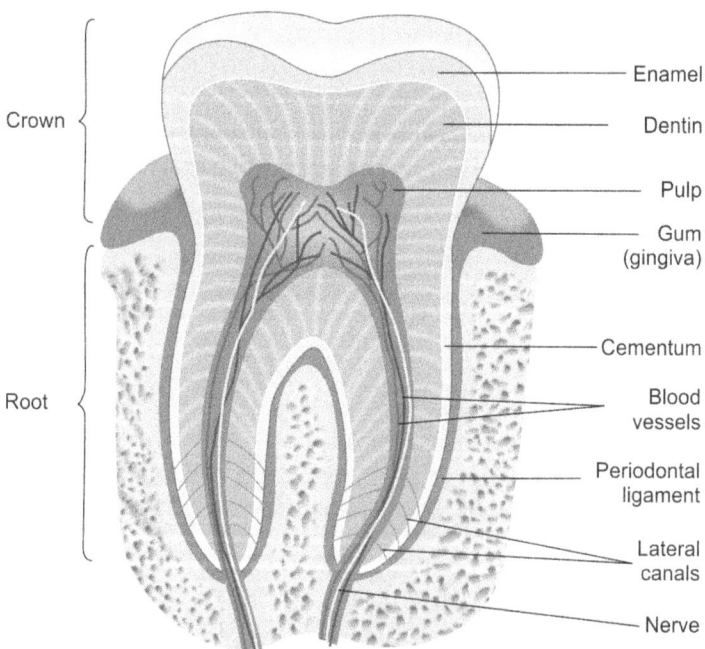

Fig. 7.5: Parts of tooth.

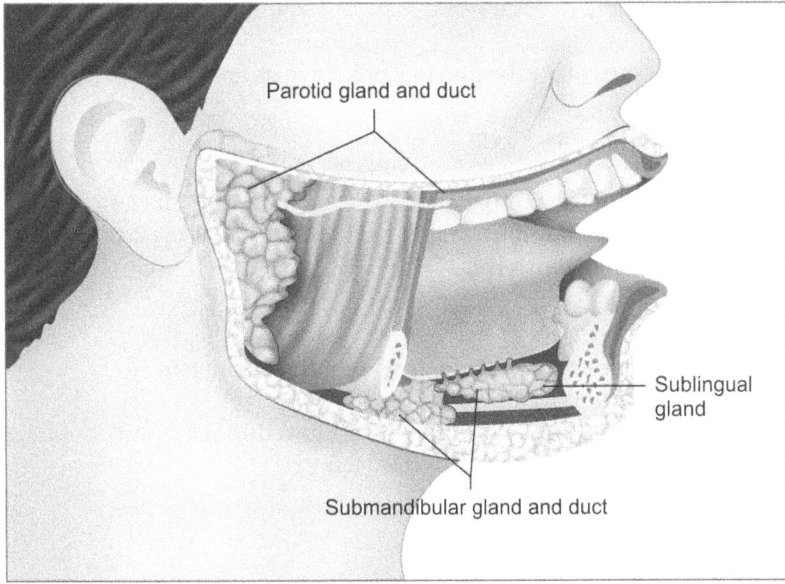

Fig. 7.6: Salivary gland.

2. **Sublingual gland:** These are situated below the tongue.
3. **Submandibular gland:** Present below the mandible.

Composition of Saliva
- Water
- Mineral salts
- Enzymes
- Lysozyme
- Immunoglobulins

Functions of Saliva
- It helps in lubrications of food
- It aids in digestion of food
- It maintains oral hygiene
- It also helps in easy swallowing of food
- It has main role in making bolus
- It gives sense of taste

Blood Supply
- **Venous drainage:** Jugular veins
- **Arterial supply:** External carotid artery

Disorders of Mouth
- **Gingivitis:** Inflammation of gums
  Glossitis: Inflammation of tongue
- **Stomatitis:** Inflammation of the mucous membrane of mouth

ESOPHAGUS

Esophagus is a muscular tube that is also known as food pipe. It runs behind the windpipe.
- **Length of esophagus:** 25 cm
- **Diameter:** 2 cm
- **It has two sphincters:** Upper and lower esophageal sphincters
- Sphincter is a circular muscle that helps in muscular constriction that is also known as peristalsis **(Fig. 7.7).**

Functions of Esophagus
- It carries food or liquid material from mouth to stomach
- It also takes part in swallowing of food
- It prevents the gastric acid reflux by contracting the lower esophageal sphincter after bolus passes into stomach.

Blood Supply
Venous drainage: Left gastric vein
Arterial supply: Esophageal arteries.

Diseases
Gastroesophageal reflux disease (GERD): In this condition, lower esophageal sphincter fails to get close and there is backflow of gastric content in esophagus.

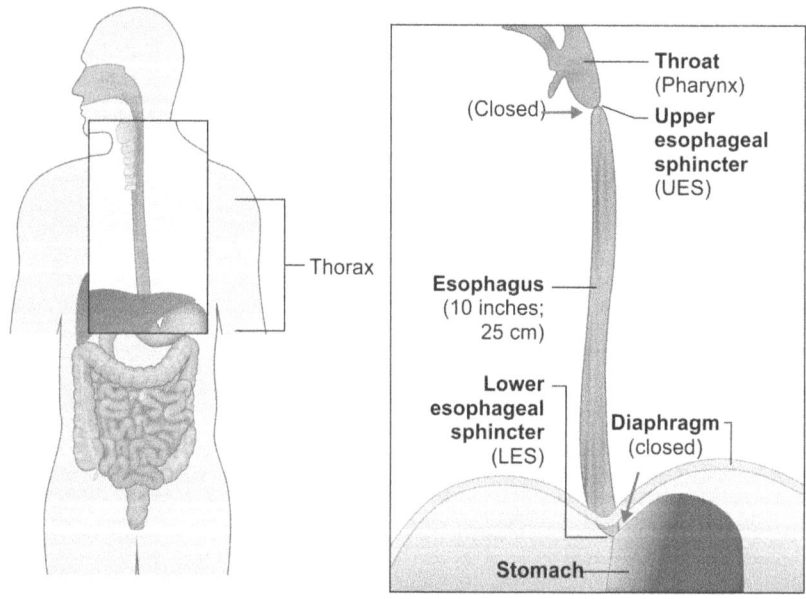

Fig. 7.7: Esophagus.

Chapter 7: Digestive System

STOMACH

- Stomach is a J-shaped organ and 25 cm long.
- It lies in left upper quadrant, umbilical, and epigastric region.
- It superiorly continues with esophagus and inferiorly connects with duodenum
- The mean capacity of stomach in an adult is 1.5–2 liter.
- Bolus gets breakdown and known as chyme in stomach (**Fig. 7.8**).

Orifices of Stomach

1. **Gastroesophageal**: It is the opening between stomach and esophagus.
2. **Pyloric**: It is the opening between stomach and duodenum.

Curvatures of Stomach

- Greater curvature
- Lesser curvature

Sphincters of Stomach

- **Cardiac sphincter:** It is also known as the lower esophageal sphincter; it closes off the top end of stomach.

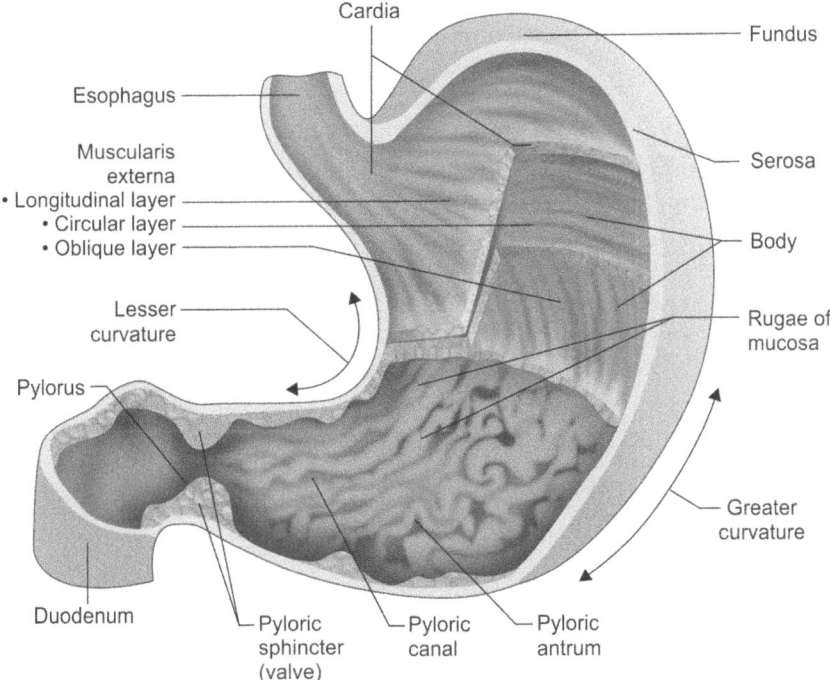

Fig. 7.8: Stomach.

- **Pyloric sphincter:** It closes off the lower end of the stomach:
  - *Rugae:* These are the gastric folds that are present in mucosal and submucosal layers of the stomach. They remain folded when the stomach is empty but as soon as the food enters the stomach, it gets flattened, and therefore these increase the surface area of the stomach.
  - *Cardia:* It surrounds the opening of the esophagus into the stomach.
  - *Fundus:* It lies above the cardia
  - *Body:* It is the largest part of the stomach.
  - *Pylorus:* It is the distal part of the stomach. It has pyloric antrum, pyloric canal, and contains pyloric sphincter.

Layers Arrangement in Stomach

All layers are same as discussed earlier about the layers of GI tract except muscular layer. It has an addition along with longitudinal and circular layer, it has oblique layer of muscles too.

Functions of Stomach

- It acts as reservoir of food
- It produces acid that is HCl, which helps in digestion and breakdown of food.
- HCl destroys the pathogens such as bacteria, viruses.
- Intrinsic factor in stomach helps in absorption of vitamin B_{12}.
- Pepsin enzyme in stomach helps in digestion of protein
- Mucin secreted by stomach protects the lining of the stomach from its own acid.

Blood Supply

- **Venous drainage:** Right and left gastric vein
- **Arterial supply:** Left gastric artery and splenic artery

Diseases

- **Peptic ulcer disease:** It is the ulcer or sore in the lining of the esophagus, stomach, and duodenum.
- **Gastritis:** Inflammation of the gastric mucosa.

PANCREAS

- Pan means all, kreas means flesh.
- It is of two types, exocrine and endocrine pancreas.
- It is a soft and elongated organ.
- It is about 15–20 cm long, 2.5–3.5 cm broad, and 1.2–1.8 cm thick.
- It weighs around 90 g **(Fig. 7.9)**.

Parts of Pancreas

- **Head:** It is situated within the curve of the duodenum
- **Neck:** It is slightly constricted part that lies between the head and body

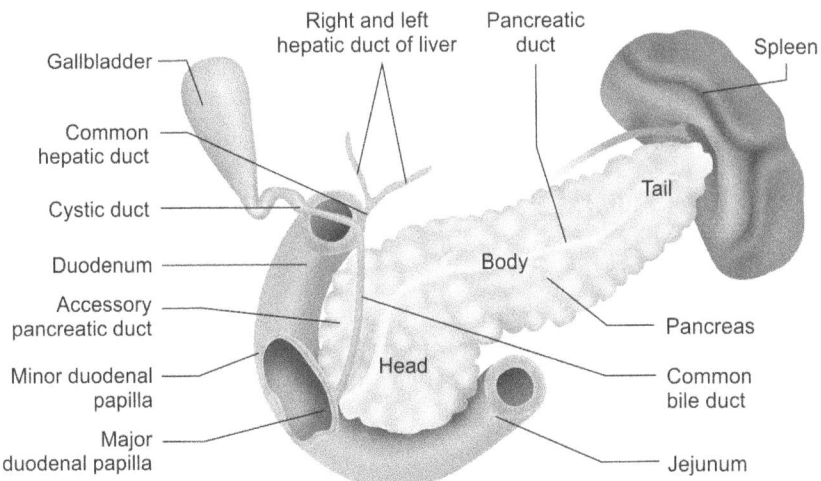

Fig. 7.9: Pancreas.

- **Body:** It is the elongated part and extends from neck till tail.
- **Tail:** It is the narrow part of the pancreas.

Types of Pancreas

1. **Exocrine:** It contains the duct through which the secretion passes. It produces pancreatic juices.
2. **Endocrine:** It is a ductless gland and secretion directly passes into the blood stream. It has four types of cells.
   a. **Alpha cells:** They produce glucagon that helps in metabolism of carbohydrate, protein and fat.
   b. **Beta cells:** They secrete the insulin; it helps in maintaining the blood glucose level of the blood.
   c. **Delta cells:** They secrete the somatostatin. It inhibits the secretion of both glucagon and insulin.
   d. **F or PP cells:** They secrete the pancreatic polypeptides.

Pancreatic Juice

- It is alkaline in nature with pH of 8-8.5
- Volume of pancreatic juice is around 500–800 mL per day.
- It contains different enzymes such as trypsinogen, chymotrypsinogen, pancreatic lipase, nucleases, and amylases.
- It is composed of 98.5% of water and 1.5% of solid.

Functions of Pancreatic Juice

- Pancreatic lipase helps in digestion of lipid
- Amylase helps in digestion of carbohydrates
- Trypsin helps in digestion of proteins.

Chapter 7: Digestive System

Blood Supply
- **Venous drainage:** Splenic and portal veins
- **Arterial supply:** Splenic artery and pancreatoduodenal artery

Disease
Pancreatitis: Inflammation of pancreas

LIVER

- It is the second largest organ after skin
- It lies mostly in right hypochondrium and epigastrium.
- In adults, it weighs around 2% of body mass.
- It is a wedge-shaped organ **(Fig. 7.10)**

Lobes of Liver
- **Right lobe:** This is the largest lobe in terms of volume.
- **Left lobe:** It is smaller than right lobe of the liver.
- **Quadrate lobe:** This lobe functionally related to left lobe.
- **Caudate lobe:** It arises from the right lobe.

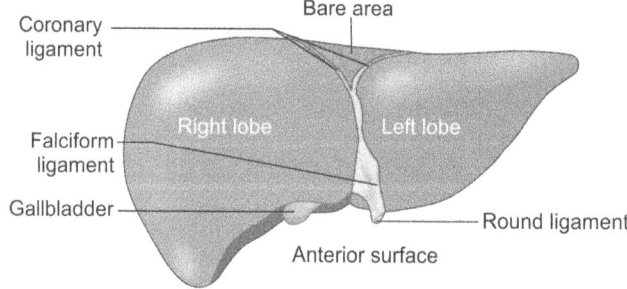

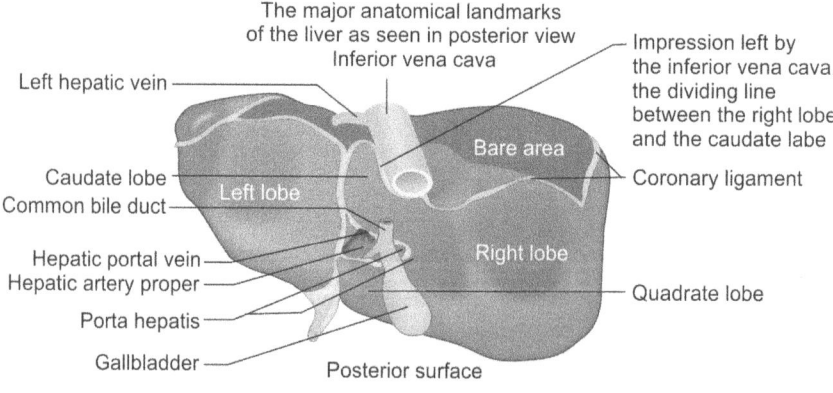

Fig. 7.10: Liver.

Attachment of Liver

Liver is attached with other viscera with the help of peritoneum folds they are such as:
- Falciform ligament
- Lesser omentum
- Coronary ligament
- Triangular ligament

Functions of Liver

- It forms and secretes the bile
- It helps in absorption of vitamins and different nutrients.
- Inactivates toxins such as alcohol.
- It synthesizes the plasma proteins such as albumin, clotting factors.
- It has Kupffer cells that participate in providing immunity by killing the disease-causing agents.

Blood Supply

- **Venous drainage:** Portal veins
- **Arterial supply:** Hepatic artery

Disease

- **Jaundice:** It is a condition in which there is the increase of bilirubin in liver causes the yellow skin, sclera, and urine.
- **Hepatitis:** It is inflammation of hepatic cells.

GALLBLADDER

- It is a pear-shaped organ
- It acts as the reservoir of bile
- It is present at the inferior surface of the liver (**Fig. 7.11**).

Parts of the Gallbladder

- **Neck:** It is the narrower part that taper into the cystic duct.
- **Body:** It is the main dilated portion of the Gallbladder.
- **Fundus:** It is the bottom portion of the liver

Functions of Gallbladder

- It stores the bile and releases in duodenum when it is required.
- It helps in regulating the concentration of bile
- It regulates the flow of bile into the duodenum.
- It responds the intestinal hormone that is cholecystokinin that contracts the Gallbladder to empty the bile from it.

Blood Supply

- **Venous drainage:** Cystic and hepatic vein.
- **Arterial supply:** Cystic artery and hepatic artery.

Chapter 7: Digestive System

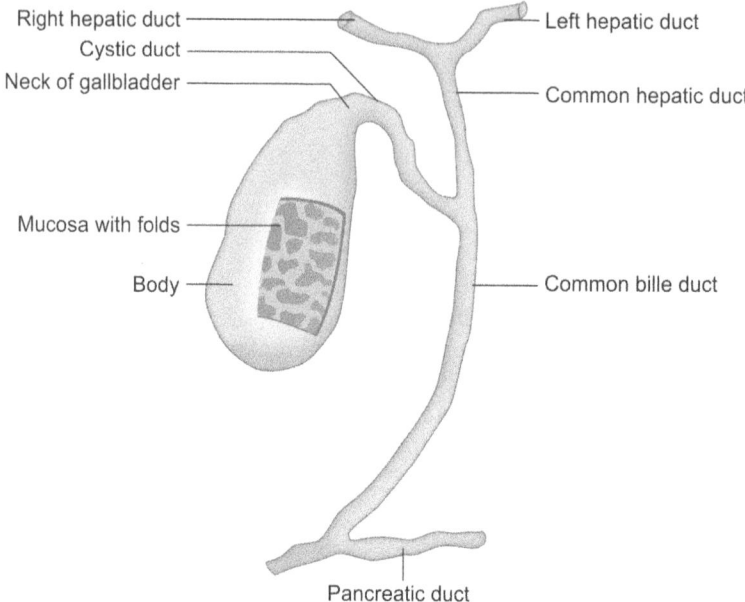

Fig. 7.11: Gallbladder.

Diseases

- **Cholelithiasis:** Stone in gallbladder
- **Choledocholithiasis:** Stone in bile duct

SMALL INTESTINE

Small intestine is divided in three main regions such as duodenum, jejunum, and ileum.

1. **Duodenum:** In Greek duodenum means 12, therefore duodenum is as long as the width of 12 fingers.
2. **Jejunum:** It is the mid portion of the small intestine; it is about 2.5 meters long. It contains the microvilli and villi these are the circular folds and increase the surface area of small intestine.
3. **Ileum:** It is the last section, and it is about 3 meters long. It absorbs mainly vitamin B_{12} and other remaining nutrients. This part connects with the first part of large intestine that is cecum with the help of ileocecal junction (Fig. 7.12).

Enzymes of Small Intestine

- **Intestinal lipase:** It helps in digestion of emulsified fat.
- **Enterokinase:** It activates trypsin which helps in breakdown of proteins.
- Other enzymes like, sucrase, maltase, and lactase help in digestion of carbohydrates

Chapter 7: Digestive System

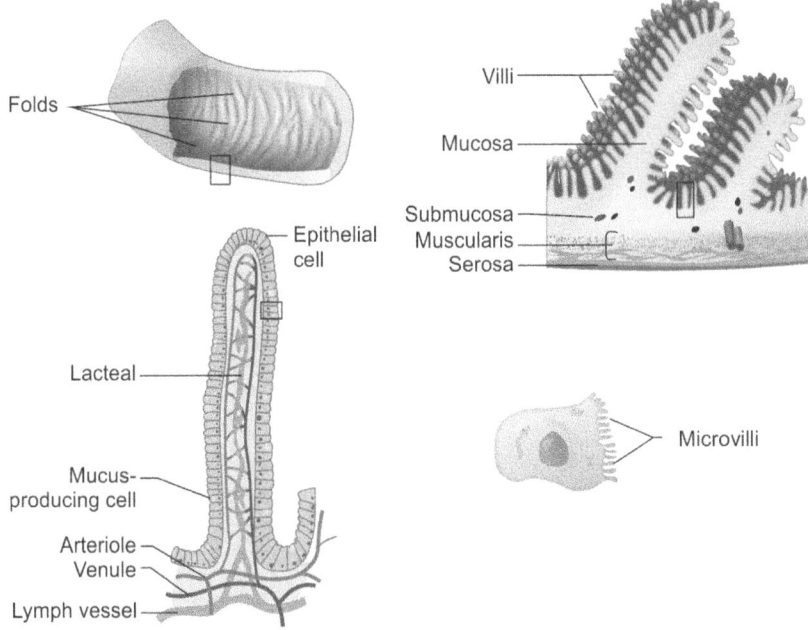

Fig. 7.12: Small intestine.

Functions of Small Intestine
- Chemical digestion completes in small intestine.
- Maximum absorption takes place in small intestine with the help of microvilli which increases the surface for better absorption.
- Secretion of hormones such as cholecystokinin (it contracts the gallbladder once food reaches the duodenum and releases the bile) and secretin (it regulates the bicarbonate secretion and maintains the alkaline environment of small intestine).

Blood Supply
- **Venous drainage:** Mesentery veins
- **Arterial supply:** Mesenteric arteries

Disease
Celiac disease: It is the condition in which immune reaction occurs due to gluten. In this condition, inflammation occurs that results in damage of the lining of small intestine.

LARGE INTESTINE

Large intestine is also known as colon and mainly divided into cecum, ascending, transverse, descending and sigmoid colon **(Fig. 7.13)**.

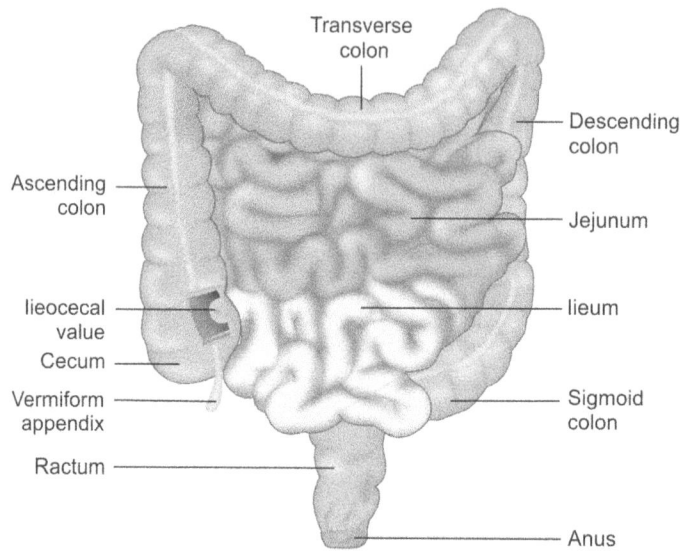

Fig. 7.13: Large intestine.

- **Cecum:** It is the proximal end part of large intestine, and it connects with end part of small intestine by meeting at ileocecal junction. Appendix is attached with the cecum, and it is about 9 cm long.
- **Ascending colon:** It extends superiorly from the right colic flexure and then turns left.
- **Transverse colon:** It extends from the right colic flexure to the left colic flexure then it turns inferiorly.
- **Descending colon:** It extends from left colic flexure of the pelvic region.
- **Sigmoid colon:** It forms an S-shaped tube and end at the rectum.

Rectum

Rectum is a muscular tube that begins at the end of the sigmoid colon, and it ends at the anal canal. It has the smooth muscles, and it is comparatively thick at the rectum in the whole digestive system.

Anal Canal

Anal canal is the last part of digestive system. It has two types of sphincters (internal and external sphincters).
1. **Internal sphincter:** It contains the smooth muscles, and it is under the control of autonomic nervous system.
2. **External sphincter:** It contains the skeletal muscles, and it is under the voluntary control.

Functions of Large Intestine

- Constitution of feces
- Helps in process of defecation

- Mass movement takes place in large intestine to pass the stool in one go in a large amount with the help of peristalsis.
- Absorption of water takes place here.
- It has goblet cells, which produces the mucus that lubricates the content.

Diseases

Hemorrhoids: It is the inflamed and swollen veins in the rectum and the anus that causes bleeding.

PHYSIOLOGY OF DIGESTION

The first phase of digestion takes place with **ingestion,** which refers to the entry of food into the alimentary canal through the mouth.

Food is chewed with the help of teeth and mixed with saliva. Saliva is secreted by salivary glands in mouth. It contains salivary amylase enzyme that helps in the digestion of carbohydrates in the food and lingual lipase, which helps in the digestion of fats. Chewing increases the surface area of the food so that digestive enzymes can act effectively. Food enters into esophagus via pharynx through mouth by the act of propulsion and includes both the voluntary process of swallowing and the involuntary process of peristalsis.

Peristalsis consists of strong, sequential, alternating waves of contraction and relaxation of alimentary wall which helps the food to move through digestive system (from up to down). Peristalsis originates by smooth muscles of alimentary canal. Peristalsis does not help in digestion but it is crucial for the movement of food particles through digestive tract.

Mechanical digestion is a physical process, which makes the food smaller to increase both surface area and mobility. It does not change the chemical nature of the food, e.g., chewing.

Food enters into stomach through cardiac sphincter. Food, which leaves the mouth, is called as bolus. In stomach mechanical churning of food takes place. It further breaks the food and exposes it to digestive juices, creating an acidic "soup" called **chyme.** In stomach, HCl provides acidic environment, which is helpful for the activation of pepsinogen to pepsin and hence digestion of protein takes place.

The chyme leaves the stomach via pyloric sphincter and reaches duodenum. Most of the digestion takes place in duodenum and small intestine. The pancreatic enzymes and bile enter into the duodenum, mixes with intestinal digestive juices, and activation of digestive enzymes take place. Here the digestion of fats, protein, and carbohydrates occurs. Pancreatic amylase pancreatic lipase, and trypsin help in the digestion of carbohydrate, fats, and proteins. The food in digestive state and mixed with all the digestive enzymes in intestine is called as **chyle.**

Chapter 7: Digestive System

SUMMARY

- Digestive system is mainly divided into two parts gastrointestinal tract and accessory organs.
- It has six basic functions such as ingestion, secretion, mixing and propulsion, chemical and mechanical digestion, absorption, and defecation.
- GI tract has four types of layers (mucosa, submucosa, muscularis, and serosa).
- Mouth is also known as oral cavity that contains a muscular tongue for swallowing and mixing of food, 16 pairs of teeth that aid in cutting, grinding and churning of food, 3 pairs of salivary glands that are parotid, sublingual and submandibular, they produce the saliva for lubrication of food.
- Esophagus is a long tube that has two upper and lower sphincters that maintain the peristalsis.
- Stomach is a J-shaped organ that churns the bolus and makes it chyme. It has rugae, which increases the surface area by getting spread when food enters the stomach.
- Small intestine has three main parts: duodenum, jejunum, and ileum. It also contains the villi and microvilli that increase the surface area, hence major absorption occurs in small intestine.
- Pancreas has exocrine and endocrine ductless gland. Exocrine secretes the pancreatic juice through pancreatic duct and endocrine secretes specialized cells that release glucagon and insulin.
- **Liver:** Largest organ that secretes the bile and has four lobes right, left lobe, caudate, and quadrate lobe.
- **Gall bladder:** It is a pear-shaped organ presents below the liver and stores the bile.
- **Large intestine:** It acts as a reservoir of feces; it has cecum, ascending, descending, transverse, and sigmoid colon. Vermiform appendix is attached with the cecum.
- Rectum is a muscular tube and anal canal is also made up of muscles and it has two sphincters internal and external.

GLOSSARY

1. **Papillae:** These are the nipple-like projections of the mucosa.
2. **Peristalsis:** It is the involuntary movements of the muscles.
3. **Sphincter:** It is the muscle that surrounds the organs of GI tract.
4. **Rugae:** Gastric rugae are the folds of mucosa and submucosa.
5. **Microvilli:** These are the finger-like projections that increase the surface area.
6. **Peritoneum:** It is the serous membrane that lines the abdominal cavity.
7. **Cadaver:** A corpse or a dead body.

LONG ANSWER TYPE QUESTIONS

1. What are the six basic processes of digestion?
2. What are the functions of stomach?
3. Describe the anatomical structure of small intestine along with labeled diagram showing villi and microvilli.

Chapter 7: Digestive System

4. Describe anatomical structure along with functions of large intestine
5. Draw labeled diagram of the following:
   a. Tongue showing papillae
   b. Tooth diagram showing all parts
   c. Stomach

MULTIPLE CHOICE QUESTIONS

1. Among these which is not an accessory organ?
   a. Liver
   b. Gallbladder
   c. Stomach
   d. Pancreas
2. Food in stomach is known as:
   a. Chyle
   b. Bolus
   c. Bile
   d. Chyme
3. What is the first part of small intestine?
   a. Ileum
   b. Duodenum
   c. Cecum
   d. Jejunum
4. What is the name of the sphincter between small and large intestine?
   a. Gastroesophageal sphincter
   b. Cardiac sphincter
   c. Ileocecal sphincter
   d. Pyloric sphincter
5. External sphincter in anal canal consists of which muscles?
   a. Skeletal
   b. Smooth
   c. Both skeletal and smooth
   d. None of the above

ANSWERS KEY

1. c   2. d   3. b   4. c   5. a

CHAPTER 8

Excretory System

INTRODUCTION

Life of every organism depends on certain basic processes. Excretion is one among them. We all obtain our nutrients from different sources, which are later digested and metabolized in our body. After metabolic reactions, the body starts to sort out useful and toxic substances in an individual. As we all know, the accumulation of the toxins may be harmful and the body removes all the metabolic wastes by the process called excretion.

Different organisms follow different modes of excretion such as kidney, lungs, skin, and eyes depending on their habitat and food habit. Aquatic animals excrete waste in the form of ammonia, while birds and insects excrete mainly uric acid. Humans produce urea as the major excretory product.

We will have a detailed look at the excretory system in human beings, different organs of the excretory system, and the mechanism of excretion in humans.

EXCRETION

The process, which is concerned with removal of nitrogeneous waste materials (e.g., urea, uric acid, CO_2, ammonia, salts, excess water, etc.) is termed excretion.

HUMAN EXCRETORY SYSTEM

The human excretory system organs include:
- A pair of kidneys
- A pair of ureters
- A urinary bladder
- A urethra

Location and Structure of Kidneys

- Mammalian kidneys are bean-shaped, reddish-brown-colored with a tough fibrous connective tissue covering called renal capsule.
- Kidneys are located laterally on either side of vertebral column levels between the last thoracic and third lumbar vertebra close to the dorsal inner wall of the abdominal cavity.
- In humans, right kidney is at slightly lower level than left kidney.
- Dorsal surface of the kidney is attached to the dorsal abdominal wall, so only its ventral surface is covered by peritoneum, therefore, this type of kidney is called **retroperitoneal kidney** or extraperitoneal kidney.

- Each kidney measures 10–12 cm in length, 5–7 cm in width, and 2–3 cm in thickness, weighing about 120–170 g in an adult.
- Lateral surfaces are convex while medial surfaces are concave.
- On the concave margins of the kidney, longitudinal opening called **hilum (hilum renalis)** is present.
- The hilum leads to a funnel-shaped space called the **renal pelvis**. The kidney tissue surrounding the pelvis is arranged in an **outer renal cortex** and inner **renal medulla**.
- The renal medulla forms conical pyramid-shaped masses, which project into the renal pelvis. These are called as **medullary pyramids or renal pyramids** (8–12 in humans).
- The cortex extends in between the medullary pyramids as renal columns called **columns of Bertini**.
- Each kidney has nearly one million complex tubular structures called **nephrons** which are the functional units. These nephrons are arranged in a radiating fashion within the renal pyramids.
- Urine produced by each nephron empties into **collecting duct**. The collecting duct passes through a **papilla** into the **renal calyx** (pleural-calyces). The renal calyces drain urine in the central cavity of renal pelvis **(Figs. 8.1A and B)**.

Postrenal Urinary Tract

Ureter

Ureter passes from the pelvis into the **ureter**. Both the ureters open through separate oblique openings into the **urinary bladder**. The obliquity of the openings prevents the backflow of urine.

Urinary Bladder

Externally, the bladder is lined by detrusor muscle; it is involuntary in nature while internally the bladder is lined by **transitional epithelium or urothelium**. This epithelium has great capacity to expand so that large volume of urine

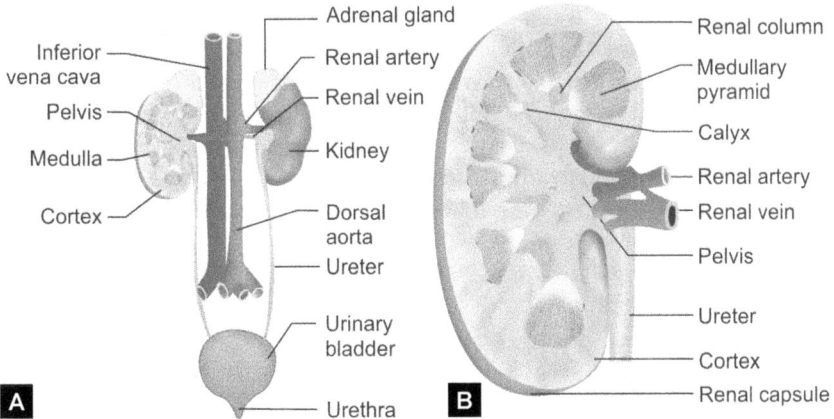

Figs. 8.1A and B: (A) Human urinary system; (B) Longitudinal section of kidney.

can be stored. Opening of urinary bladder is controlled by sphincters made of circular muscles. In humans, two sphincters are present:
1. Inner = Internal sphincter (made up of involuntary muscle)
2. Outer = Outer sphincter (voluntary muscle)

Urethra

Urinary bladder opens into a membrane duct called **urethra**. In females, both sphincters are present in membranous urethra.

- **Passage of urine:** Nephron → Collecting duct → Duct of Bellini → Papilla → Renal calyx → Renal pelvis → Ureters → Urinary bladder → Urethra
- **Micturition:** The process of release of urine is called micturition and the neural mechanism causing it is called micturition reflex. This reflex is initiated when interoceptors present in the wall of urinary bladder, get stimulated by the tension created due to stretching of bladder wall as the bladder gradually fills with urine brought into it by the ureters.

  In response, the stretch receptors on the walls of the bladder send signals to the central nervous system (CNS). The CNS passes on motor messages to initiate the contraction of smooth muscles of the bladder and simultaneous relaxation of urethral sphincter causing the release of urine.

Structure of Nephron

- Nephron is the structural and functional unit of kidney. It is an epithelial tube, which is about 3 cm long and 20–60 µm in diameter.
- A nephron can be divided into following regions **(Fig. 8.2)**:
    - *Bowman's capsule:* At the proximal or closed end the nephron is expanded and curved inwardly to form a double-walled cup-shaped Bowman's capsule. It is formed by the afferent arteriole (a fine branch of renal artery).
        - Malpighian body: Glomerulus and its surrounding Bowman's capsule together forms Malpighian body or renal corpuscle. It is responsible for the first step of urine formation (filtration).

        The outer wall of Bowman's capsule is composed of flattened squamous cells. The inner, invaginated wall that lines the concavity of Bowman's capsule is composed of a special type of cells called **Podocytes**, which are arranged in an intricate manner so as to leave some minute spaces called **filtration slits** or slit pores. These cells are actually simple squamous cells and bear finger-like projections, which are coiled around the capillaries of glomerulus.

        The Bowman's capsule is followed by a short neck part lined by ciliated cuboidal epithelium.
    - *Proximal convoluted tubule (PCT):* The epithelial cells of this region are specialized for transport of salts and other substances from the lumen to the interstitial fluid. The membranes of these cells facing the tubule lumen have numerous microvilli (finger-like projections or Brush Borders), which increase the surface area.

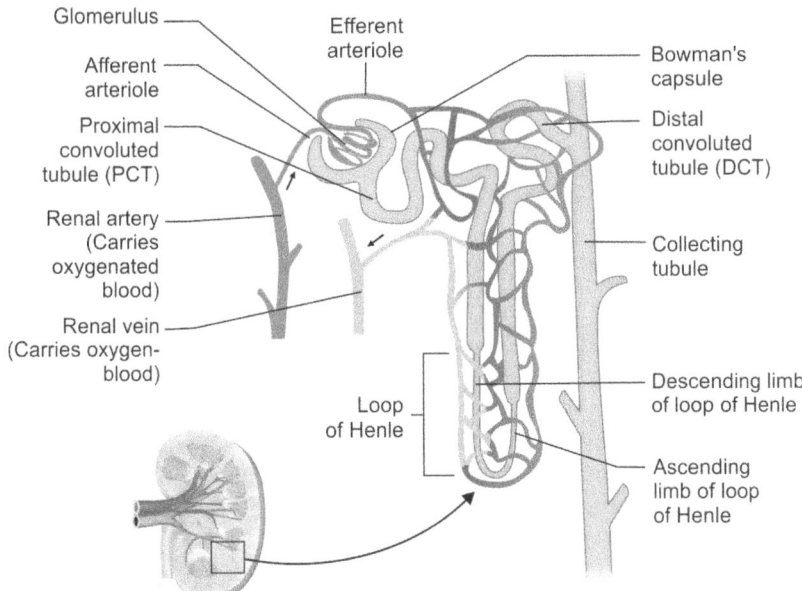

Fig. 8.2: Structure of nephron.

- *Loop of Henle:* It starts after the PCT and ends before the distal convoluted tubule (DCT).
    - Descending limb: Its upper part constitutes thick segment:
        - Has the same diameter as PCT
        - Is also lined by simple cuboidal epithelium
    - Its lower part constitutes thin segment:
        - Is lined by flat squamous cells
    - Ascending limb: Its upper part constitutes thick segment:
        - Has the same diameter as DCT
        - Is also lined by simple squamous epithelium
      Its lower partconstitutes thin segment:
        - Is lined by flat squamous cells
- *Distal convoluted tubule (DCT):* The ascending limb of Henle's loop merges into DCT. This is lined by cuboidal epithelial cells. The DCT of different nephrons open into a straight tube called **collecting duct.** Collecting ducts (present in medullary pyramids) are long tubules, which traverse through the medulla in the pyramids.
  All ducts of Bellini then open at the tip of the papillae into the pelvis.
    - Renal cortex: The malpighian corpuscle, PCT, and DCT of the nephrons are located here.
    - Renal medulla: Loop of Henle, collecting duct, and ducts of Bellini are found in this region.

TABLE 8.1: Comparison between cortical and juxtamedullary nephrons.	
Cortical nephrons	**Juxtamedullary nephrons**
Malpighian corpuscles are located close to the kidney surface	Malpighian corpuscles are located at the junction of cortex and medulla
Their loop of Henle is mostly confined to cortex and a very small part of it runs in the medulla	The loop of Henle of these nephrons is long, dipping deep down into the medulla
Peritubular capillary network is present	Peritubular capillary network is not well developed
Vasa recta is absent or highly reduced	Vasa recta present

Types of Nephron
There are two types of nephron (**Table 8.1**):
1. **Cortical nephron:** These are the nephrons present within the cortex.
2. **Juxtamedullary nephron:** These have long loops of Henle and extend into the medulla. These are about 20%.

MECHANISM OF URINE FORMATION
It involves three steps or processes:
1. Ultrafiltration or glomerular filtration
2. Selective tubular reabsorption
3. Tubular secretion

Ultrafiltration or Glomerular Filtration
It is the primary step in urine formation. Glomerular filtration occurs as blood passes into the glomerulus producing a plasma-like filtrate (minus proteins) that gets captured by the Bowman's (glomerular) capsule and funneled into the renal tubule (**Fig. 8.3**). Glomerular filtration rate (GFR) in a healthy individual is approximately **125 mL/min, i.e., 180 L/day.**

On an average, 1,100–1,200 mL of blood is filtered by the kidneys per minute (renal blood flow), which constitute roughly 20–25% of the blood pumped by each ventricle of the heart in a minute (cardiac output) and of this blood 650 mL is the blood plasma (55%). This 650 mL is called **renal plasma flow (RPF).**

Selective Tubular Reabsorption
As the filtrate travels along the length of the nephron, the cells lining the tubule selectively, and often actively, take substances from the filtrate and move them out of the tubule into the blood.

This includes very physiologically important molecules such as water, sodium, chloride, and bicarbonate (along with many others) as well as molecules that the digestive system used a lot of energy to absorb, such as glucose and amino acids. These molecules would be lost in the urine, if not reclaimed by the tubule cells. These cells are so efficient that they can reclaim all of the glucose and amino acids and up to 99% of the water and important

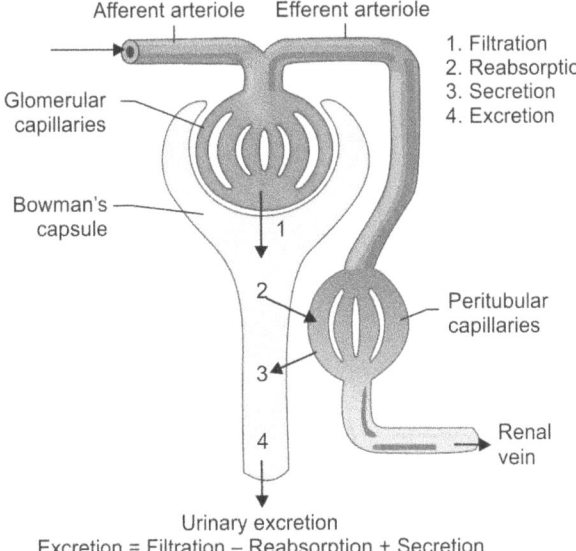

Fig. 8.3: Glomerular filtration.

ions lost due to glomerular filtration. The filtrate that is not reabsorbed becomes urine at the base of the collecting duct **(Fig. 8.4)**.

Tubular Secretion

These substances secreted into the tubule are destined to leave the body as components of urine **(Table 8.2)**.

Chemical Composition of Urine

95% = water
2% = salts
2.7% = urea
0.3% = other materials (drugs, Hippuric acid, Uric acid, Vitamin-C, and dyes)
- An adult human excretes on an average 1–1.5 L of urine per day.
- Urine is pale yellow in color due to urochrome pigment.
- On an average, 25–30 g of urea is excreted out per day.
- Normal urine is slightly acidic (pH = 6.0)

REGULATION OF KIDNEY FUNCTION

- **Regulation involving hypothalamus:** Antidiuretic hormone (ADH) can also cause constriction of blood vessels resulting in an increase in the blood pressure thereby increasing the blood flow in the glomerulus and glomerular filtration rate.
- **Regulation involving juxtaglomerular apparatus (JGA):** Regulation by JGA is known as renin-angiotensin mechanism. It causes vasodilation and decreases blood pressure in the blood vessels. The ANF mechanism provides the necessary check to the renin-angiotensin mechanism **(Fig. 8.5)**.

Chapter 8: Excretory System

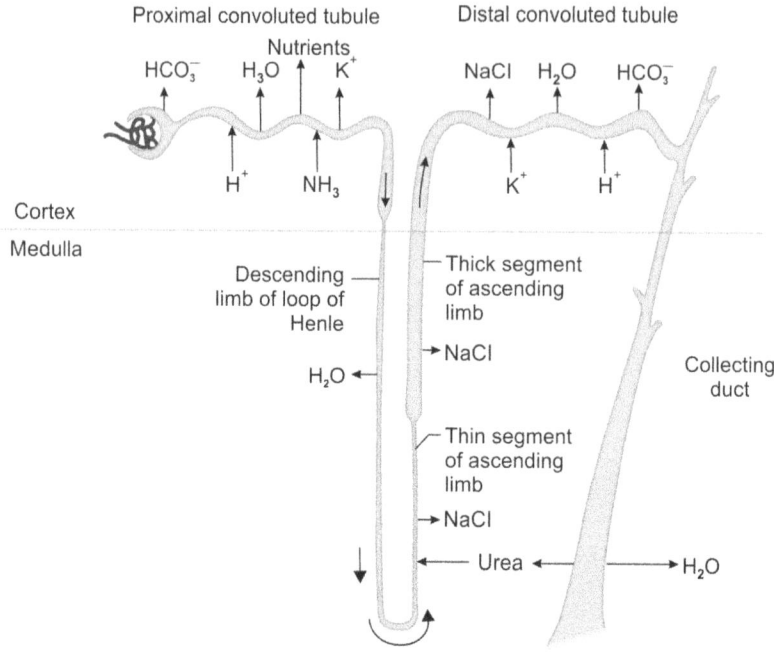

Fig. 8.4: Reabsorption and secretion of major substances at different parts of the nephron. (Arrows indicates direction of movement of materials).

TABLE 8.2: Substances secreted or reabsorbed in the nephron and their locations.				
Substance	**PCT**	**Loop of Henle**	**DCT**	**Collecting ducts**
Glucose	Almost 100% reabsorbed; secondary active transport with Na+			
Oligopeptides, proteins, amino acids	Almost 100% reabsorbed; symport with Na+			
Vitamins	Reabsorbed			
Lactate	Reabsorbed			
Creatinine	Secreted			
Urea	50% reabsorbed by diffusion; also secreted	Secretion, diffusion in descending limb		Reabsorption in medullary collecting ducts; diffusion

Contd...

Contd...

Substance	PCT	Loop of Henle	DCT	Collecting ducts
Sodium	65% actively reabsorbed	25% reabsorbed in thick ascending limb; active transport	5% reabsorbed; active	5% reabsorbed, stimulated by aldosterone; active
Chloride	Reabsorbed, symport with Na$^+$, diffusion	Reabsorbed in thin and thick ascending limb; diffusion in ascending limb	Reabsorbed; diffusion	Reabsorbed; symport
Water	67% reabsorbed osmotically with solutes	15% reabsorbed in descending limb; osmosis	8% reabsorbed if ADH; osmosis	Variable amounts reabsorbed, controlled by ADH, osmosis
Bicarbonate	80–90% symport reabsorption with Na$^+$	Reabsorbed, symport with Na$^+$ and antiport with Cl$^-$; in ascending limb		Reabsorbed antiport with Cl$^-$
H$^+$	Secreted; diffusion		Secreted; active	Secreted; active
NH$_4^+$	Secreted; diffusion		Secreted; diffusion	Secreted; diffusion
HCO$_3^-$	Reabsorbed; diffusion	Reabsorbed; diffusion in ascending limb	Reabsorbed; diffusion	Reabsorbed; antiport with Na$^+$
Some drugs	Secreted		Secreted; active	Secreted; active
Potassium	65% reabsorbed; diffusion	20% reabsorbed in thick ascending limb; symport	Secreted; active	Secretion controlled by aldosterone; active
Calcium	Reabsorbed; diffusion	Reabsorbed in thick ascending limb; diffusion		Reabsorbed, if parathyroid hormone present; active
Magnesium	Reabsorbed; diffusion	Reabsorbed in thick ascending limb; diffusion	Reabsorbed	
Phosphate	85% reabsorbed, inhibited by parathyroid hormone, diffusion		Reabsorbed; diffusion	

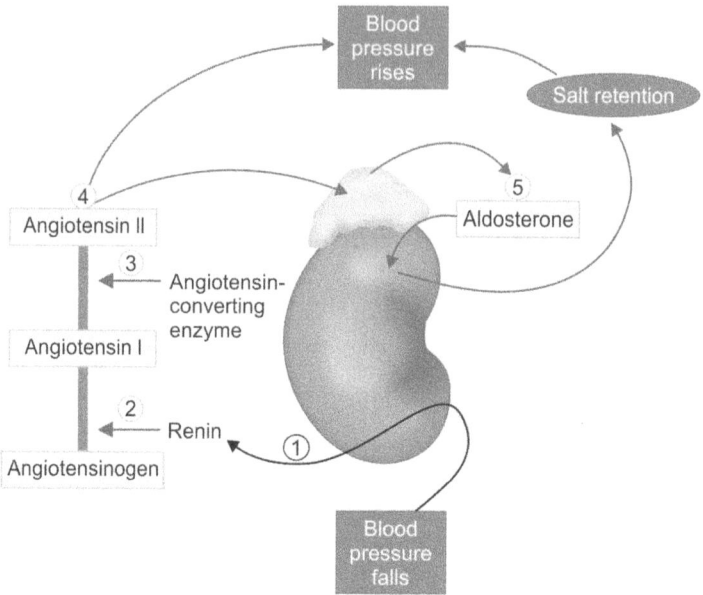

Fig. 8.5: Regulation of kidney function.

ROLE OF OTHER ORGANS IN EXCRETION

- **Lungs:** Human lungs eliminate **around 200 mL/min** of CO_2 and about 400 mL of water per day in normal resting condition.
- **Skin:** Humans possess two types of glands in skin:
    1. *Sweat glands:* These excrete sweat. Sweat contains 99.5% water, NaCl, lactic acid, small amount of urea, amino acid, and glucose.
    2. *Sebaceous glands:* These secrete sebum, which contain waxes, sterols, other hydrocarbons, and fatty acids. This secretion provides a protective oily covering the skin.
- **Liver:** Liver is the main site for elimination of cholesterol, bile pigments (bilirubin and biliverdin), degraded steroid hormones, some vitamins, and drugs.

DISORDERS OF THE EXCRETORY SYSTEM

- **Uremia:** Malfunctioning of kidneys can lead to accumulation of urea in blood, a condition called uremia, which is highly harmful and may lead to kidney failure. In such patients, urea can be removed by a process called **hemodialysis**. As nitrogenous wastes are absent in the dialyzing fluid, these substances freely move out, thereby clearing the blood. The cleared blood is pumped back to the body through a vein after adding antiheparin to it. This method is a boon for thousands of uremic patients all over the world.
- **Renal failure:** It is a syndrome characterized by urea dysfunction, oliguria, and anuria, sudden rise in metabolic waste products like urea and creatinine in blood (uremia).
    It is either of acute or chronic nature.

Chapter 8: Excretory System

- **Renal calculi:** Formation of stones within kidney. These calculi are made of calcium phosphate, uric acid, cysteine, or calcium oxalate.
- **Glomerulonephritis:** Inflammation of glomeruli of kidney.

EXCRETION AND ITS IMPORTANCE

They are in a leaf cell, which allows vacuoles to crystallize. We usually see the vacuoles get filled, and then the leaf drops. These are known as **excretophores**. Saps and gums are also the types of excretion displayed by plants, which we see with our naked eye.

Sweat also helps in bringing down the temperature of the body because high temperatures can be fatal or cause life-threatening injuries.

Unicellular organisms like amoeba also produce metabolic waste products and they rid themselves of these by a process called diffusion. But they also use this as a method for respiration since they obtain oxygen through this process.

SUMMARY

- Excretion is the physiological process of elimination of metabolic waste from the body. Though excretion in human beings takes place through lungs, skin, liver, and kidneys, they are the main organs of the human excretory system. They are bean-shaped organs, which weigh between 120 and 170 g and their length ranges from 10 to 12 cm.
- The major functions of the kidneys are to:
  - Maintain the body's pH
  - Reabsorption of nutrients
  - Regulates blood pressure
  - Excretion of wastes from the body
  - Removal of excess fluid from the body
  - Secret hormones that help in the production of red blood cell, acid regulation, etc.
- The functional unit of the kidney is the nephron. Each kidney consists of millions of nephron, which plays a significant role in the filtration and purification of blood. The nephron is divided into two portions, namely, the glomerulus and the renal tubule and helps in the removal of excess waste from the body.
- There are two types of nephrons—cortical nephrons and juxtamedullary nephrons.
- The mechanism of urine formation involves three steps or processes:
  1. Ultrafiltration or glomerular filtration
  2. Selective tubular reabsorption
  3. Tubular secretion
- The kidney glomerulus filters blood mainly based on particle size to produce a filtrate lacking cells or large proteins. The tubule cells remove them from the blood and secrete them into the filtrate, thereby removing them from the body.
- The entire volume of the blood is filtered through the kidneys about 300 times per day, and 99% of the water filtered is recovered. Reabsorption reclaims most filtered substances in the PCT in association with active transport of sodium.
- The regulation of kidney function occurs through the involvement of hypothalamus and juxtaglomerular apparatus.

Chapter 8: Excretory System

GLOSSARY

1. **Excretion:** Elimination or removal of waste products or toxic products from the body.
2. **Kidney:** Kidney is bean-shaped, reddish brown colored organ which is located laterally and retroperitoneally on either side of the vertebral column.
3. **Retroperitoneal:** The area behind the peritoneum or outside the peritoneal cavity.
4. **Hilum:** The concave margin of kidney, longitudinal opening called hilum.
5. **Nephron:** Nephron is the basic functional unit of kidney.
6. **Glomerular filtration rate:** It is the rate at which the blood is filtered from the kidney and forms filtrate. Normal GFR is 125 mL/min.
7. **Selective reabsorption:** The physiologically important molecules are reabsorbed into the blood capillaries.
8. **Tubular secretion:** This is the secretion of the substances into the kidney tubules so that they can be eliminated via urine.

LONG ANSWER TYPE QUESTIONS

1. Explain the structure of kidney with diagram.
2. Describe the various sections of nephron.
3. Write about the mechanism of urine formation.
4. Write down the regulation of kidney function involving juxtaglomerular apparatus (JGA).
5. Describe the role of liver, lungs, and skin in excretion.

SHORT ANSWER TYPE QUESTIONS

1. What is micturition?
2. Define glomerular filtration rate (GFR).
3. What is hemodialysis?
4. Write the location of kidneys present in human body.
5. Differentiate between cortical and juxtamedullary nephrons.

MULTIPLE CHOICE QUESTIONS

1. Bowman capsule is located in:
   a. Cortex   b. Henle's loop
   c. Bladder   d. None
2. A notch present on the medial side of kidney is known as:
   a. Ureter   b. Pelvis
   c. Hilus   d. Pyramid
3. In cortex area of kidney, all structures are found, *except*:
   a. Bowman capsule   b. DCT
   c. Majority of collecting duct   d. Malpighian body
4. Functional and structural unit of kidney is:
   a. Nephron   b. Seminiferous tubule
   c. Acini   d. None

Chapter 8: Excretory System

5. The blood vessel supplying blood into Bowman's capsule is:
   a. Afferent arteriole
   b. Efferent arteriole
   c. Renal vein
   d. Renal portal vein
6. Podocytes are present in:
   a. Afferent arteriole
   b. Efferent arteriole
   c. Peritubular network
   d. Bowman's cup
7. Difference between glomerular filtrate and plasma is of:
   a. Proteins
   b. Potassium
   c. First is white whereas later is yellow
   d. First is yellow whereas later is white
8. The hormone that produces reabsorption of water from glomerular filtrate is:
   a. Oxytocin
   b. Vasopressin
   c. Relaxin
   d. Calcitonin
9. Kidney stone is produced due to:
   a. Deposition of sand particles
   b. Precipitation of proteins
   c. Crystallization of oxalates
   d. Blockage of fat
10. Hemodialysis helps patients with:
    a. Uremia
    b. Anemia
    c. Diabetes
    d. Goiter

ANSWERS KEY

1. a   2. c   3. c   4. a   5. d
6. a   7. b   8. c   9. a   10. a

CHAPTER 9

Nervous System

NERVOUS SYSTEM

The nervous system is the control center of our body. All bodily activities, voluntary, and involuntarily, are controlled by the nervous system. The response by nervous system is very quick and life-saving. The nervous system consists of brain, spinal cord, and nerves. It detects and responds to changes that are taking place inside and outside the body. This chapter deals with the nervous system, parts and their function.

CENTRAL NERVOUS SYSTEM

The central nervous system (CNS) is responsible for higher neural functions such as memory, learning, emotions, touch, motor skills, vision, breathing, temperature, hunger, and every process that regulates body.

The CNS consists of two major interconnected organs:
1. The brain
2. The spinal cord

The Brain

The brain is situated within the cranial cavity. It is protected by cranial bone. Weighs about 3 pounds in adults. The parts of brain include (**Fig. 9.1**):
A. **Forebrain**
   i. Cerebrum
   ii. Diencephalon
B. **Midbrain**

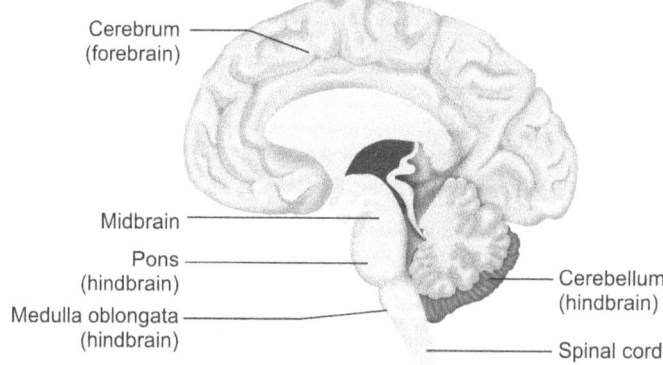

Fig. 9.1: The brain.

C. **Hindbrain**
   i. Pons	ii. Medulla	iii. Cerebellum

Forebrain

Cerebrum

- It is the largest part of the brain and is composed of hemispheres on the right and left.
- It performs greater functions such as touch, vision, and hearing interpretation as well as speech, reasoning, emotions, learning, and fine movement control.
- The brain is divided into two halves—the hemispheres on the right and left.
- A bundle of fibers called the corpus callosum joins them, which transmits messages from one side to the other.
- Each hemisphere controls the opposite side of the body. If a stroke occurs on the right side of the brain, left arm or leg may be weak or paralyzed.
- In general, the left hemisphere controls speech, comprehension, arithmetic, and writing. The right hemisphere controls creativity, spatial ability, artistic, and musical skills (**Fig. 9.2**).

Lobes of the Brain

- There are separate fissures in the cerebral hemispheres, dividing the brain into lobes.
- There are four lobes in each hemisphere: frontal, temporal, parietal, and occipital.

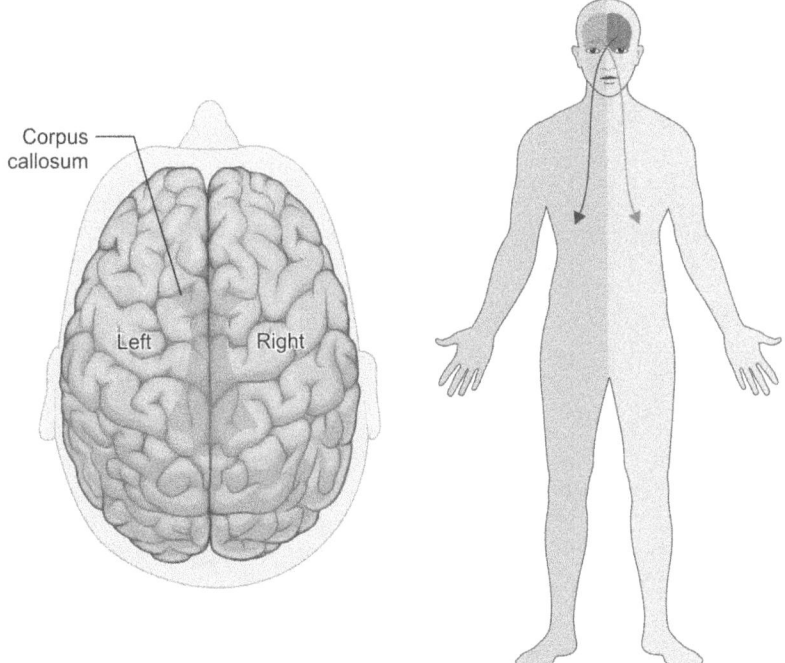

Fig. 9.2: Cerebrum.

Once again, each lobe may be split into areas that serve very specific functions. There are very complicated interactions between the brain lobes and between the right and left hemispheres (**Fig. 9.3**).

Gyri: The entire surface of the cerebral hemispheres exhibits elevated ridges of tissue called gyri, separated by shallow grooves called **sulci**.

Fissures: Less numerous are the deeper grooves of tissue called fissures, which separate large regions of the brain (**Fig. 9.4**).

Diencephalon

* The diencephalon, or interbrain, sits atop the brain stem and is enclosed by the cerebral hemispheres.

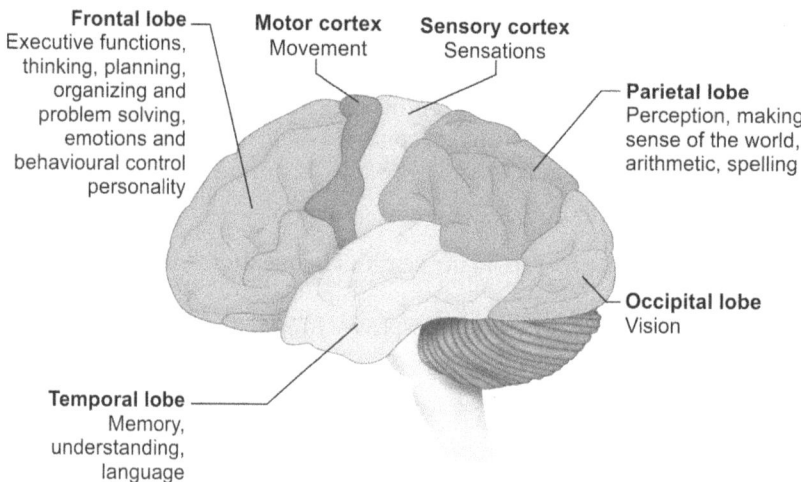

Fig. 9.3: Lobes of brain.

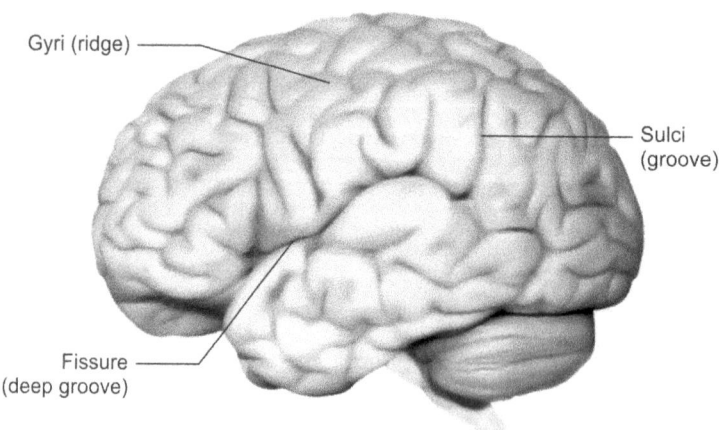

Fig. 9.4: Gyri and fissure.

- **Thalamus:** The thalamus is a relay station for sensory impulses passing up to the sensory cortex, enclosing the shallow third ventricle of the brain.
- **Hypothalamus:** The hypothalamus is the diencephalon floor; it is an important center of autonomic nervous system because it plays a role in regulating body temperature, water balance, and metabolism. It is also the center of many drives and emotions, and as such it is an important part of the so-called limbic system or emotional-visceral brain **(Fig. 9.5)**.

Hindbrain

Pons: The pons is a rounded structure just below the midbrain, and this region of the brain stem is mainly fiber tracts. However, there are substantial nuclei involved in breathing regulation.

Medulla oblongata: The lower portion of the brain stem is the medulla oblongata; it contains nuclei that regulate essential visceral activities; it contains centers that control, among others, heart rate, blood pressure, breathing, swallowing, and vomiting.

Cerebellum: From under the occipital lobe of the cerebrum, the broad, cauliflower-like cerebellum projects dorsally.

Structure: Like the brain, there are two hemispheres and a convoluted surface of the cerebellum; it also has an external cortex composed of gray matter and an inner area of white matter.

Function: The cerebellum provides skeletal muscle movement with precise timing and regulates our balance equilibrium

Coverage: Fibers reach the cerebellum from the equilibrium apparatus of the inner ear, the eye, the proprioceptors of the skeletal muscles and tendons, and many other areas **(Fig. 9.6)**.

Meninges

The meninges are the membrane covering the brain and the spinal cord. The meninges consist of three membranes:

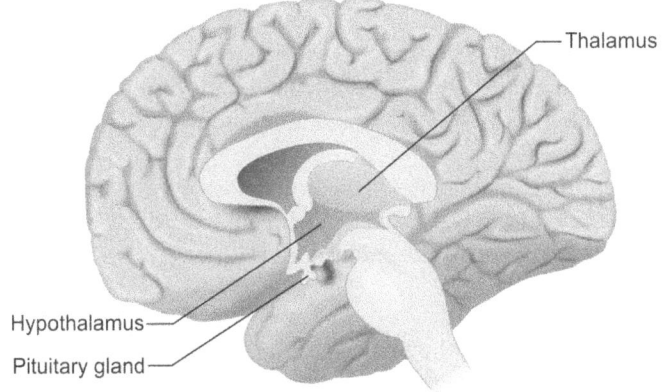

Fig. 9.5: Importance of diencephalon.

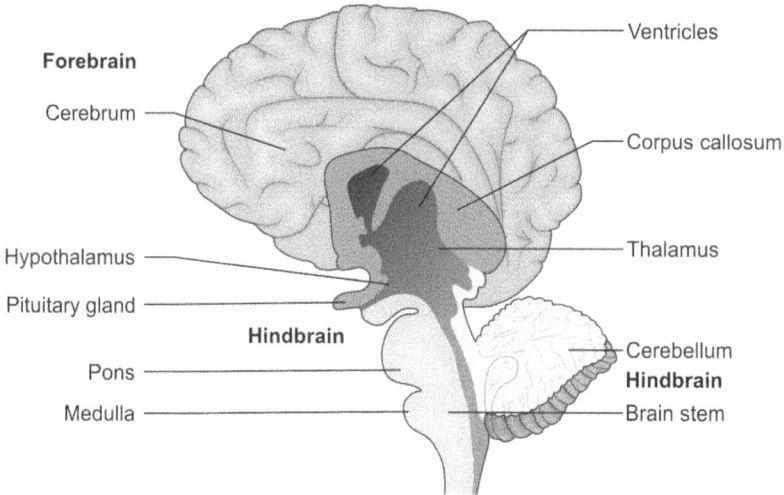

Fig. 9.6: Parts of brain.

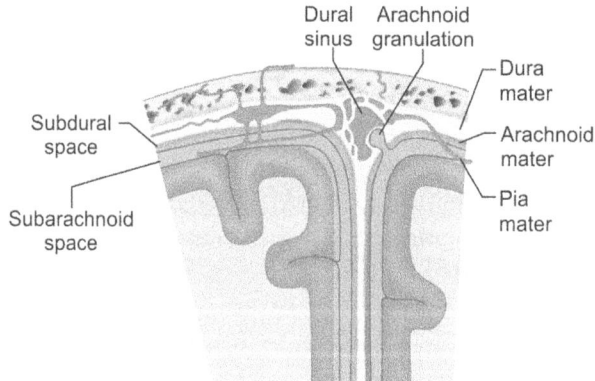

Fig. 9.7: Membranes of meninges.

1. **The dura mater:** Dura mater is the outer layer of the meninges. It consists of two layers of fibrous tissue.
2. **The arachnoid mater:** The arachnoid mater is the middle layer of meninges that present between the dura mater and pia mater. It is a layer of fibrous tissue.
3. **The pia mater:** The pia mater is the innermost layer of the meninges that adhere to the brain. It is formed of a delicate layer of connective tissue. It runs downward covering the spinal cord **(Fig. 9.7)**.

Ventricles

There are four ventricles in the brain that contains cerebrospinal fluid. These are the irregular-shaped cavities present within the brain. The ventricles of the brain are:

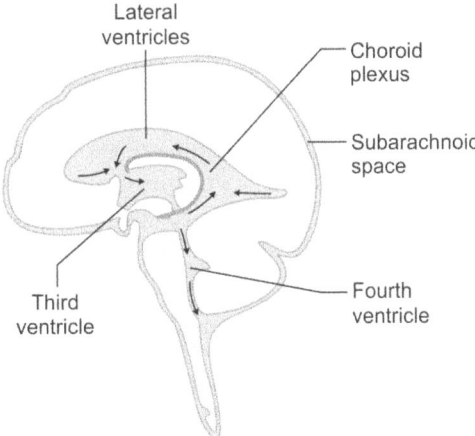

Fig. 9.8: Ventricles.

- **Two lateral ventricles:** The lateral ventricles are present one on each within the cerebral hemispheres below the corpus callosum. There are right and left ventricle.
- **Third ventricle:** The third ventricle is present below the lateral ventricles. The cerebral aqueduct is the canal that connects the third ventricle to the fourth ventricle.
- **Fourth ventricle:** Fourth ventricle is a diamond-shaped cavity present below the third ventricle. It lies between the pons in front and the cerebellum at the back. The cerebrospinal fluid from the third ventricle drains through the cerebral aqueduct into the fourth ventricle **(Fig. 9.8)**.

Cerebrospinal Fluid

Cerebrospinal fluid (CSF) is a watery substance similar to blood plasma, from which it forms.
- **Contents:** The CSF contains less protein and more vitamin C, and glucose.
- **Choroid plexus:** CSF is continually formed from blood by the choroid plexuses; choroid plexuses are clusters of capillaries hanging from the "roof" in each of the brain's ventricles.
- **Function:** The CSF in and around the brain and cord forms a watery cushion that protects the fragile nervous tissue from blows and other trauma.
- **Normal volume:** CSF forms and drains at a constant rate so that its normal pressure and volume (150 mL about half a cup) are maintained.
- **Lumbar tap or lumber puncture:** The CSF sample for testing is obtained by a procedure called lumbar tap or lumber puncture. The withdrawal of fluid for testing decreases CSF fluid pressure. Therefore, the patient must remain in a horizontal position (lying down) for 6–12 hours after the procedure to prevent an agonizingly painful "spinal headache".

The Spinal Cord
- Spinal cord begins from the brainstem.

Chapter 9: Nervous System

- It also has the ability to produce instructions, i.e., reflexes, but only for spontaneous processes.
- The primary role is to pass on information between the CNS and the periphery.
- The spinal cord is a long, delicate structure of a tube that starts at the end of the stem of the brain and goes down almost to the bottom of the spine.
- Nerves that carry incoming and outgoing signals between the brain and the rest of the body consist of the spinal cord.
- The spine is composed of 33 individual back bones in most adults (vertebrae).
- Much like the skull covers the brain, the spinal cord is covered by vertebrae.
- Disks made of cartilage, which serve as cushions, separate the vertebrae, minimizing the forces produced by movements such as walking and jumping.
- Like the brain, the spinal cord is covered by three layers of tissue (meninges). The spinal cord and meninges are contained in the spinal canal, which runs through the center of the spine.
- The spinal cord is about 43 cm long in adult women and 45 cm long in adult men and weighs about 35–40 grams. It lies within the vertebral column, the collection of bones (back bone) **(Fig. 9.9)**.

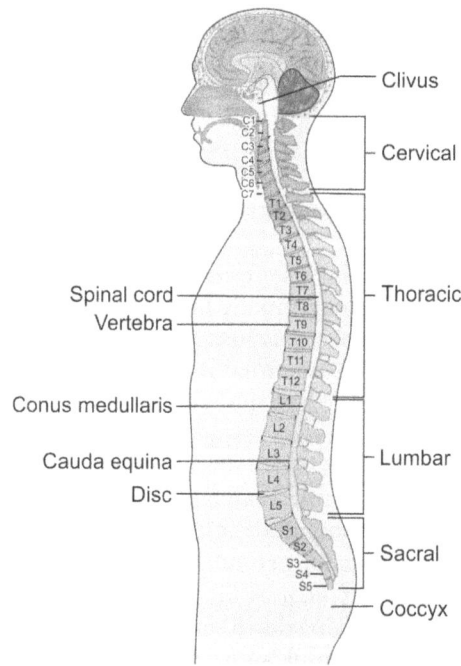

Fig. 9.9: Spinal cord.

PERIPHERAL NERVOUS SYSTEM

* Peripheral nervous system (PNS) is made up of all the nerves that lead into and out of the CNS **(Fig. 9.10)**.
* **Functional divisions:**
  ➢ Somatic nervous system
  ➢ Autonomic nervous system; sympathetic, parasympathetic, and enteric divisions

  The peripheral nervous system is made up of two parts **(Fig. 9.11)**:
  1. Somatic nervous system (SNS)
  2. Autonomic nervous system
     * The sympathetic nervous system
     * The parasympathetic nervous system
     * The enteric nervous system

  The peripheral nervous system consists of:
  ➢ Twelve pairs of cranial nerves that arise from the brain.
  ➢ Thirty one pairs of spinal nerves that emerge from the spinal cord.
* The somatic nervous system consist of sensory neurons that convey information from cutaneous and special sense receptors primarily in the head, body wall, and extremities to the CNS and motor neurons from the CNS that conduct impulses to skeletal muscles only.

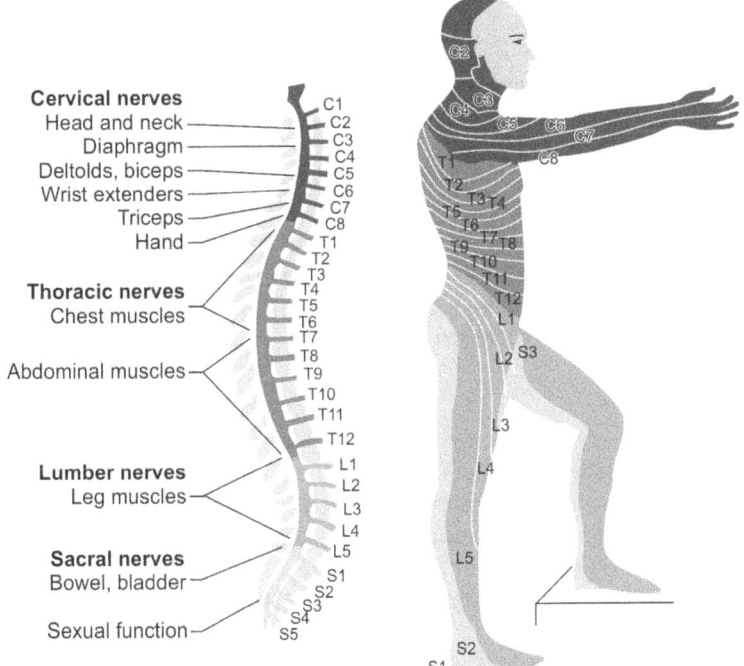

Fig. 9.10: Peripheral nervous system.

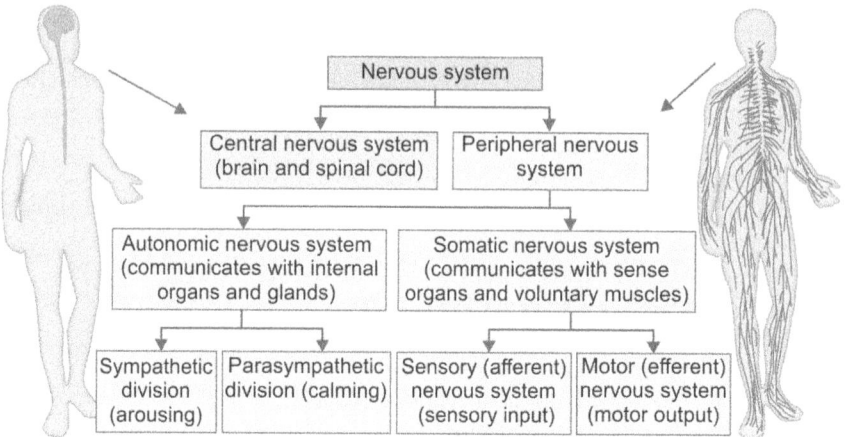

Fig. 9.11: Parts of peripheral nervous system.

Spinal Nerves

- There are 31 pairs of spinal nerves. They emerge from the spinal cord and leave the vertebral canal by passing through the intervertebral foramen.
- They are grouped according to the region of the vertebra from where it leaves the spinal cord on both sides of the vertebral column.
- There are:
  - Cervical nerves—8
  - Thoracic nerves—12
  - Lumbar nerves—5
  - Sacral nerves—5
  - Coccygeal nerves—1
- Each spinal nerve is connected to the spinal cord by a dorsal root and a ventral root. The cell bodies of the sensory neurons are in the dorsal root ganglion, but the motor neuron cell bodies are in the gray matter. The two roots join to form the spinal nerve just before the nerve leaves the vertebral column. Because all spinal nerves have both sensory and motor components, they are all mixed nerves.

Cranial Nerves

- The cranial nerves are composed of 12 pairs of nerves that stem from the nervous tissue of the brain (**Table 9.1**).
- Some nerves have only sensory component, some only a motor component and some have both components.
- MNEMONICS to remember the cranial nerves:
  "Old Own Olympus, Tiny Tops, A French And German, Views Some Hopes"

AUTONOMIC NERVOUS SYSTEM

- The autonomic nervous system, also referred to as the efferent nervous system, provides motor impulses to the smooth muscle and glandular

TABLE 9.1: Cranial nerves and their functions.

#	Name	General function	Specific function
I	Olfactory	Sensory	Olfaction
II	Optic	Sensory	Vision
III	Oculomotor	Motor	Eyeball muscles
IV	Trochlear	Motor	Eyeball muscle
V	Trigeminal	Both	S—Face and oral cavity M—Muscles of mastication
VI	Abducens	Motor	Eyeball muscle
VII	Facial	Both	S—Taste from anterior 2/3rd of tongue M—Muscles of facial expression
VIII	Vestibulocochlear	Sensory	Audition Equilibrium
IX	Glossopharyngeal	Both	S—Taste from posterior 1/3rd of tongue M—Pharyngeal muscles
X	Vagus	Both	Viscera
XI	Accessory	Motor	Sternocleidomastoid and trapezius
XII	Hypoglossal	Motor	Tongue muscles

Pneumonic to learn cranial nerves name
Pneumonic to learn the general function of cranial nerves

epithelium of the heart muscle. The autonomic nervous system regulates many processes of the body, such as breathing, digestion, sweating, and shivering.
* Autonomic nervous system controls involuntary or automatic functions, the autonomic nervous system has two parts: the **sympathetic nervous system** and the **parasympathetic nervous system (Fig. 9.12)**.
* The **sympathetic nervous system** prepares the body for sudden stress. When something frightening happens, the sympathetic nervous system makes the heart beat faster so that it sends blood quickly to the different body parts that might need it. It also causes the adrenal glands at the top of the kidneys to release adrenaline, a hormone that helps give extra power to the muscles for a quick getaway. This process is known as the body's "fight or flight" response.
* The **parasympathetic nervous system** does the exact opposite: It prepares the body for rest. It also helps the digestive tract move along body can efficiently take in nutrients from the food.

NERVE TISSUE

* The nervous system consists of a large number of cells known as neuron.
* Each neuron has a cell body, axon and dendrites. The neurons are supported by a special type of connective tissue called neuroglia.

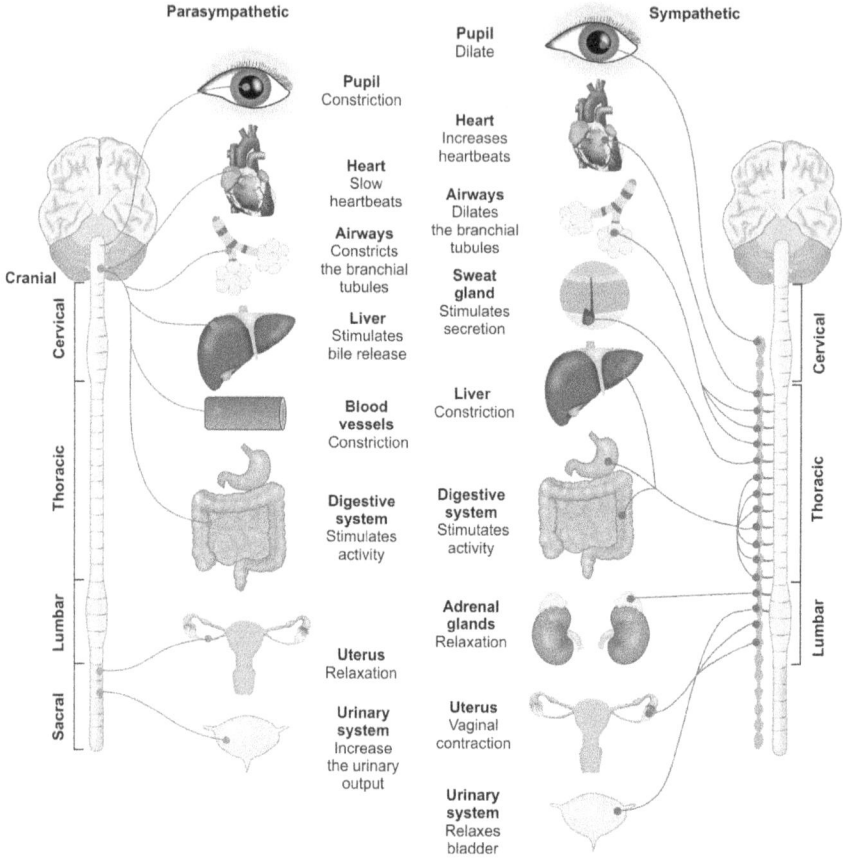

Fig. 9.12: Sympathetic and parasympathetic nervous system.

- Neurons conduct nerve impulses. The nerve impulse or the action potential is the physiological unit of the nervous system.
- The bundle of axons bound together called nerves. Neurons do not divide and it requires continuous supply of oxygen and glucose for its survival.
- The neurons have the properties of irritability and conductivity.
- Irritability is the ability to initiate a nerve impulse and conductivity is the ability of neuron to transmit nerve impulse.
- **Cell body:** The nerve cell bodies forms the gray matter of the nervous system. They are present at the periphery of the brain and at the center of the spinal cord. The group of cell bodies are called nuclei in the central nervous system and ganglia in the peripheral nervous system.
- **Axon:** A single branch (in most neuron), which conducts nerve impulses away from the cell body. Myelin sheath and neurilemma are coverings
- **Dendrites:** Thin branching extensions of the cell body. They are short processes that have the same structure as that of the axon **(Fig. 9.13)**.

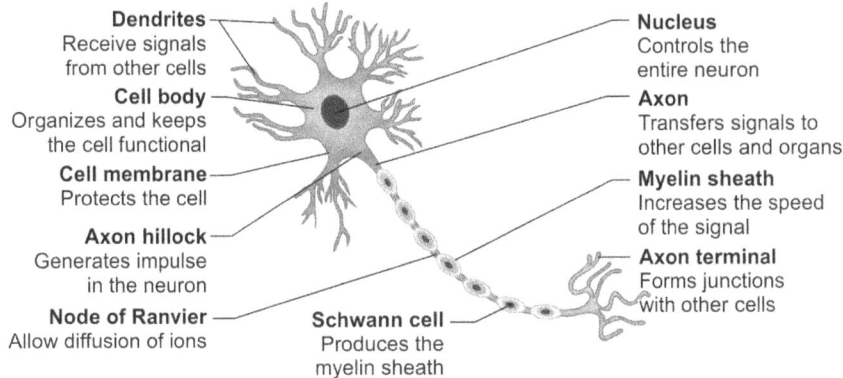

Fig. 9.13: Parts of neuron.

SUMMARY

- **Nervous system:** The nervous system consists of brain, spinal cord, and nerves.
- It detects and responds to changes that are taking place inside and outside the body.
- **Central nervous system (CNS):** The central nervous system is responsible for higher neural functions such as memory, learning, emotions, touch, motor skills, vision, breathing, temperature, hunger, and every process that regulates body.
- The central nervous system consists of two major interconnected organs: **The brain and the spinal cord.**
- **The brain consists of three parts:** Forebrain (cerebrum, diencephalon), midbrain, hindbrain (pons, medulla, cerebellum).
- **Lobes of the brain:** The cerebral hemispheres have distinct fissures, which divide the brain into lobes. Each hemisphere has four lobes—frontal, temporal, parietal, and occipital.
- **Meninges:** The meninges are the membrane covering the brain and the spinal cord. The meninges consist of three membranes—the dura mater, the arachnoid mater, the pia mater.
- **Ventricles:** There are four ventricles in the brain that contains cerebrospinal fluid, two lateral ventricles, third ventricle, fourth ventricle.
- The CSF in and around the brain and cord forms a watery cushion that protects the fragile nervous tissue from blows and other trauma (150 mL—about half a cup)
- The spinal cord is a long, fragile tube-like structure that begins at the end of the brainstem and continues down almost to the bottom of the spine. The spinal cord consists of nerves that carry incoming and outgoing messages between the brains.
- **The peripheral nervous system consist of:** Somatic nervous system and autonomic nervous system (the sympathetic nervous system and the parasympathetic nervous system).
- **Cranial nerves:** The cranial nerves are composed of 12 pairs of nerves that stem from the nervous tissue of the brain. Olfactory, optic, oculomotor, trochlear, trigeminal, abducent (or abducens), facial, vestibulocochlear, glossopharyngeal, vagus, accessory, and hypoglossal.
- Each neuron has a cell body, axon and dendrites. The neurons are supported by a special type of connective tissue called neuroglia.
- Neurons conduct nerve impulses. The nerve impulse or the action potential is the physiological unit of the nervous system

Chapter 9: Nervous System

GLOSSARY

1. **Brain:** The organ inside the head that controls thought, memory, feelings, and activity.
2. **Central nervous system:** The main system of nerve control in a living thing, consisting of the brain and the main nerves connected to it.
3. **Cerebrospinal fluid:** CSF circulates throughout the brain and spinal cord.
4. **Cerebrum:** Largest part of the brain; responsible for voluntary muscle activity, vision, speech, taste, hearing, thought, memory.
5. **Cranial nerves:** Twelve pairs of nerves that carry messages to and from the brain with regard to the head and neck (except the vagus nerve).
6. **Dendrite:** Microscopic branching fiber of a nerve cell that is the first part to receive a nerve impulse.

LONG ANSWER TYPE QUESTION

1. Explain the structure and function of the neurons.

SHORT ANSWER TYPE QUESTIONS

1. Draw a well label diagram of brain.
2. Explain the cranial nerves and its functions.
3. Explain the functions of nerve cells.
4. Write down the short note on the following:
   a. CSF
   b. Hypothalamus and its function
   c. Lobes of the brain and its function

MULTIPLE CHOICE QUESTIONS

1. What is the basic unit of the nervous system?
   a. Glial cell
   b. Meninges
   c. Neurons
   d. Cerebrospinal fluid
2. The neuron cell is made of the following parts?
   a. Axon
   b. Dendrite
   c. Nucleus
   d. All the above
3. Which of the following is the correct order of meninges from the inner side?
   a. Pia mater – arachnoid mater – dura mater
   b. Pericardium – myocardium – endocardium
   c. Dura mater – pia mater – arachnoid mater
   d. Duro mater – arachnoid mater – pia mater
4. In the left hemisphere, Broca's area is related to_____.
   a. Speech
   b. Smell sensation
   c. Impulses received from eyes
   d. Reasoning and learning
5. Space, which separates arachnoid mater and dura mater is _____.
   a. Epidural
   b. Mediastinum
   c. Subdural
   d. Subarachnoid

ANSWERS KEY

1. c   2. d   3. d   4. a   5. c

Chapter 9: Nervous System

ATLAS

Identify and label the diagrams.

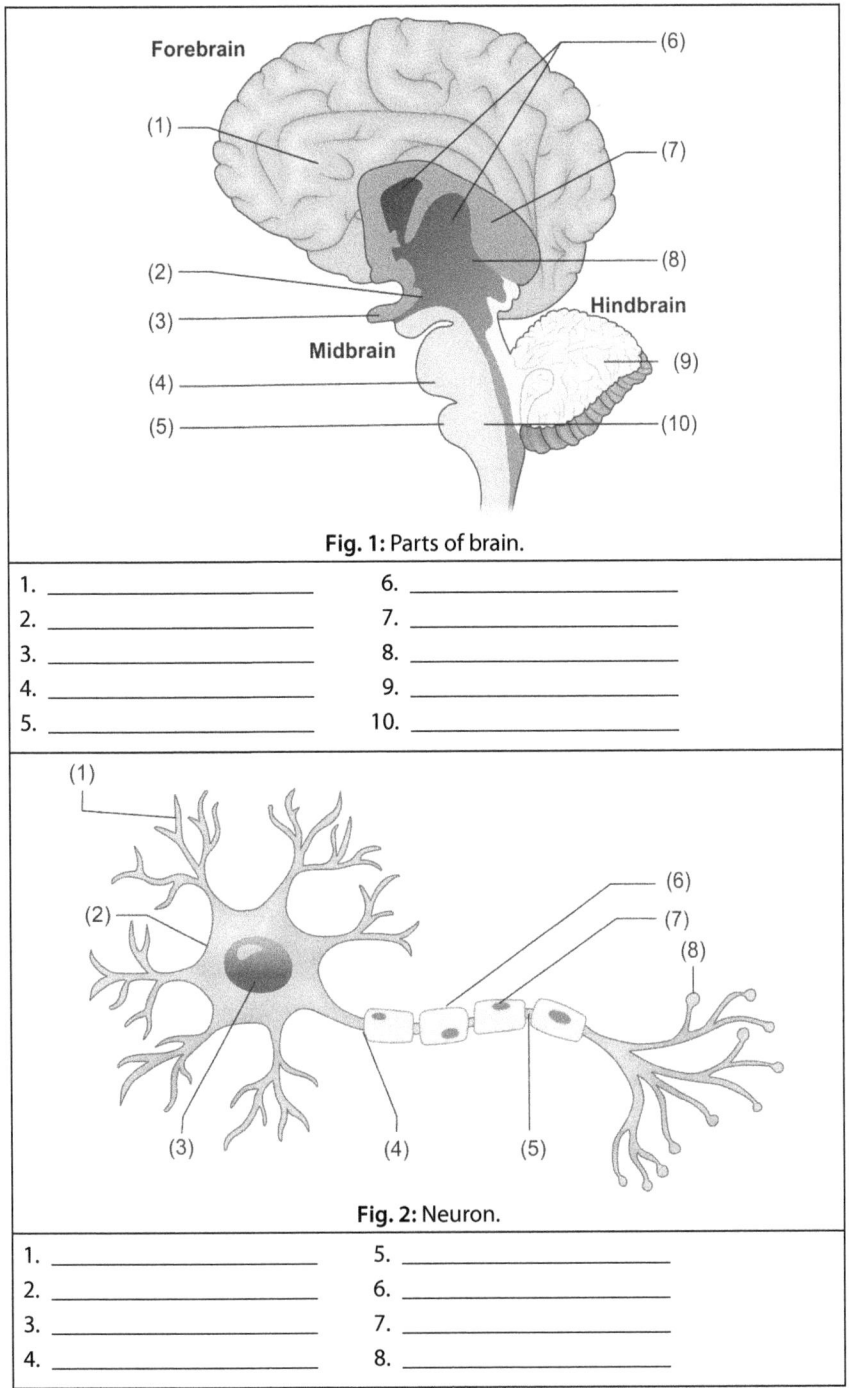

Fig. 1: Parts of brain.

1. _____   6. _____
2. _____   7. _____
3. _____   8. _____
4. _____   9. _____
5. _____   10. _____

Fig. 2: Neuron.

1. _____   5. _____
2. _____   6. _____
3. _____   7. _____
4. _____   8. _____

CHAPTER 10

Sense Organs

INTRODUCTION

We have heard about the five senses. These senses help us to see, taste, hear, touch, and smell. The sense organs responsible for the sensations are eye, tongue, ear, skin, and eyes.

This chapter helps us to understand how the sense organs work their location and their function.

Introduction to Sense Organs

"Sense organs are the organs that react on outer stimuli by sending impulses to the sensory nervous system".

As we all have heard about the five senses, i.e., see, hear, smell, taste, and touch. We use our eyes to see, we use ears to hear, we use nose to smell, to taste we use our tongue, and we touch with the help of our skin. So basically, human beings have five sense organs, i.e., eyes, ear, nose, tongue, and skin (**Fig. 10.1**).

Five types of sensory receptors—the type of stimuli they detect:

1. **Mechanoreceptors:** Mechanoreceptors involved in movement and balance.
2. **Thermoreceptors:** Skin which respond to external internal temperature.
3. **Pain receptors:** Stimulated by lack of O_2, chemicals form by damaged cells and inflammatory cells.
4. **Chemoreceptors:** Detect changes in levels of O_2, CO_2, and H^+ ions (pH) as well as chemicals that stimulate taste and smell receptors.
5. **Photoreceptors:** It responds to light falling on it.

Special Senses

- Vision, hearing, taste, and smell General (somesthetic, somatosensory)
- Receptors widely distributed in skin, muscles, tendons, joints, and viscera
- It recognize touch, pressure, stretch, heat, cold, and pain
- **Vision:** Eye
- **Hearing:** Ear
- **Equilibrium:** Ear
- **Taste:** Taste receptors
- **Smell:** Olfactory system general senses
- **Skin:** Hot, cold, pressure, pain

Chapter 10: Sense Organs

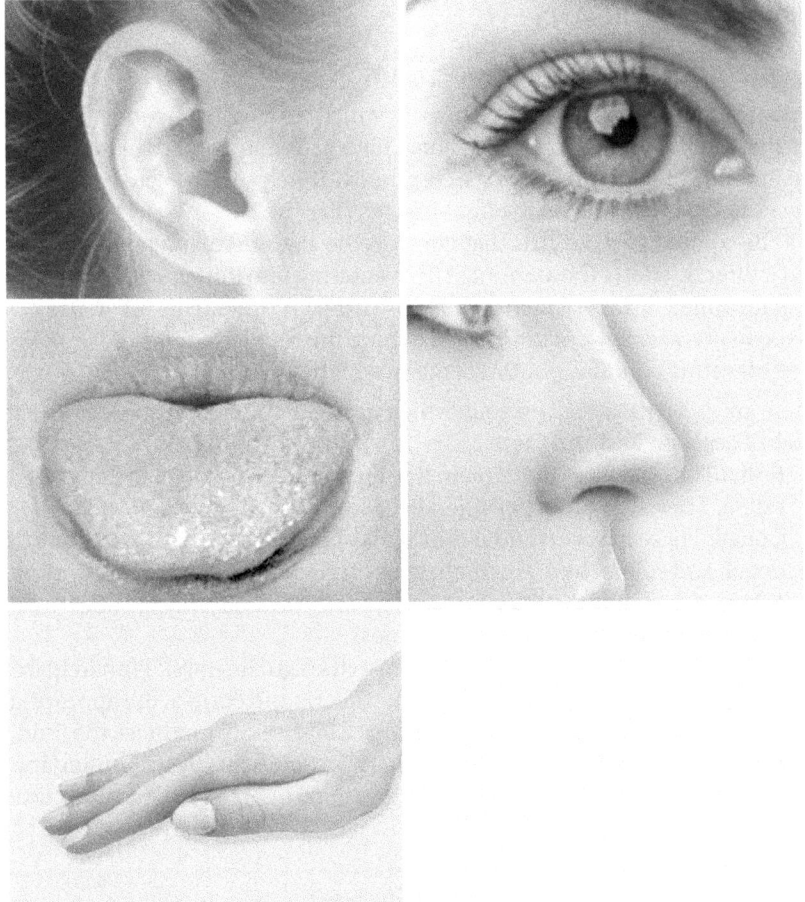

Fig. 10.1: Sense organs.

- **Muscles, joints, and tendons:** Stretch receptors respond to stretch or compression
- **Pain receptors:** Somatic or visceral

WHAT ARE THE SENSE ORGANS?

Sense organs provide the required sense for semantics through various organs and a network of nerves in response to a particular physical process. These senses govern our interaction with the environment.

We have five sense organs namely:
1. Eyes
2. Ears
3. Nose
4. Tongue
5. Skin

FIVE SENSE ORGANS

Eyes—Sight or Ophthalmoception

Eyes are known as visual sensory organs, which we have in our body. These are sensitive to light images. The eyes may have different color depending upon the amount of melanin present in our body. It helps in the sense of sight by detecting and focusing on the light images (**Fig. 10.2**).

The colored part, i.e., iris that controls the size and diameter of the pupil, and it directly affects the amount of light entering into the eyes. It has a gel-like structure filled inside it which is called as vitreous humor. This substance gives shape to the very back of the eyeball, where the retina is found.

This retina contains photoreceptors, which detect light.

There are two types of cell present, which perform functions distinct from each other. These are Rod and Cones.
1. **Rods:** These sensors function in low light and are found at the edge of the retina. They also aid in peripheral vision.
2. **Cones:** These types of retinal cells works best in bright light, detecting fine detail, and color. There are three types of cones for detecting three primary colors of light, namely, blue, red and green. When any one of cones are not present, it usually cause color blindness.

Vision occurs when light enters the eye through the pupil. With help from other important structures in the eye, like the iris and cornea, the appropriate amount of light is directed toward the lens. Ciliary body produces the fluid in the eye called aqueous humor. While ciliary muscle helps in accommodation. Where aqueous humor is a gel-like structure filled between the lens and cornea

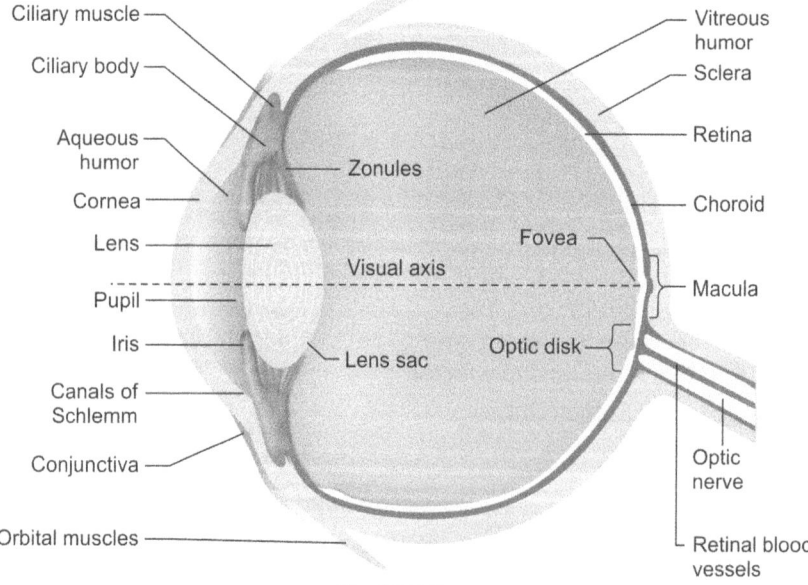

Fig. 10.2: Eye.

and vitreous humor is filled between the back surfaces of the lens to the front surface of the retina. We can see every structure of eyes has their own role. Eye functions with the help of all these structures.

Ears—Hearing or Audioception

Ears are considered as auditory organs of our body. They help us to hear sounds. Our auditory system detects vibrations in the air and this is how we hear the sounds.

The ears have three sections, i.e., inner ear, the middle ear, and the outer ear. All sounds are basically vibrations, so the outer ear transfers these vibrations into the ear canal, where these vibrations are transformed by the brain into meaningful sound. Apart from hearing, this senses also important for balancing our body or equilibrium (**Fig. 10.3**).

- **Parts:** Tympanic cavity, auditory ossicles, muscles of the ossicles
- **Function:** Transforming a high-amplitude low-force sound wave into a low-amplitude high-force vibration and transmitting it to the internal ear
- **Parts:** Bony labyrinth (vestibule, semicircular canals, cochlea) and membranous labyrinth (utricle, saccule, semicircular ducts, cochlear duct)
- **Function:**
  ➤ Bony labyrinth supports its membranous counterparts
  ➤ Utricle and saccule provide information about the position of the head
  ➤ Semicircular ducts provide information about movements of the head
  ➤ Cochlear duct provides hearing information

Tongue—Taste or Gustaoception

The tongue helps in perceiving various tastes and flavors. The taste buds are present between the papillae on the tongue—these help in sensing different tastes.

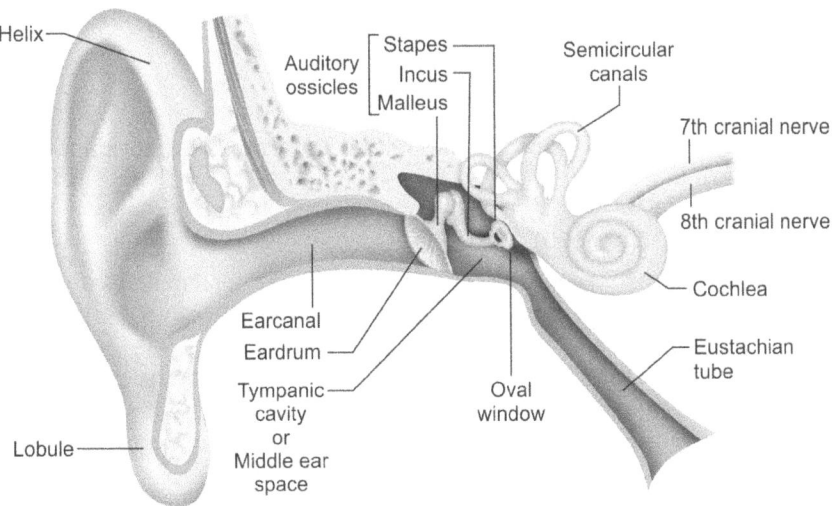

Fig. 10.3: Ears.

Senses of taste and smell kind of work together. If you cannot smell something, you cannot even taste it. The sense of taste is gustaoception.

Chemoreceptors in the nose works in detecting any kind of smell, and there are four different types of taste buds which helps to detect different types of tastes like sweetness, sourness, bitterness, and saltiness.

Skin—Touch or Tactioception

Skin is the largest organ of our body. It comes in sense of touch, which is also considered as tactioception.

The skin has its general receptors that can recognize touch, pain, pressure, and temperature. They are present all over the skin. These skin receptors generate an impulse, and when its active it is carried to the brain and then to the spinal cord.

Nose—Smell or Olfalcoception

The nose is an olfactory organ. And this system helps us recognize different smells. This sense of organ also aids our sense of taste. The sense of smell is also known as olfaction.

As one breathes in, the air enters into the nasal cavity. The olfactory cells are the chemoreceptors, which means that the olfactory cells have protein receptors that can detect the differences in the chemicals. These chemicals bond up to cilia, which conducts a **nerve impulse** and is carried to the brain. The brain then translates these impulses into a meaningful smell. During a cold, the body produces mucus and that affects and block the sense of smell; this is ultimately hinders the taste of our food and it tastes bland.

OTHER SENSORY ORGANS

Other than these five sense organs, there are another two organs, which help orienting us with the world. And it helps maintain our body posture.
1. Maintaining our body balance.
2. Stabilize our head and body during movement.
3. Identifying the orientation and posture of our bodies in relation to the environment. The vestibular system is useful in ordinary movement and equilibrium.

Proprioception System

This system is described as the position of joints. This system helps the body to identify the muscles, joints, and limbs located in 3D space and the direction it is moving in relation to the body.

Walking or kicking without looking at our feet, balancing on one leg, touching the nose with eyes closed and the ability to sense the surface on which we are standing upon, are a few examples of proprioception system.

Sensation Receptors

The size of the stimulus can affect the number of receptors that respond, and the strength of the stimulus can affect how much they respond. For example,

Chapter 10: Sense Organs

when a puppy sits on your lap, a big number of receptors respond to the puppy's weight, warmth, claws, and the vibrations from it.

SUMMARY

The nervous system is used for sensing the external and internal position of an organism, and for inducing muscle movement. Human sensation is achieved by the stimulation of specialized neurons, organized into five different modalities—touch, balance, taste, smell, hearing, and vision. Touch includes pressure, vibration, temperature, pain, and itch.

GLOSSARY

1. **Eyes:** These are visual sensory organs of our body.
2. **Rods:** These sensors function in low light and are found at the edge of the retina. They aid in peripheral vision.
3. **Cones:** The type of retinal cells work best in bright light. Helps in detecting color and fine details.
4. **Ear:** Ears are considered as auditory organs of our body.
5. **Skin:** Skin is the largest organ of our body which helps in tactioception.

LONG ANSWER TYPE QUESTIONS

1. Which is the most sensitive sense organ and why?
2. Which neurons receive information from sensory organs?
3. How do sensory organs send signals to the brain?
4. How does a stimuli trigger sense?

SHORT ANSWER TYPE QUESTIONS

1. Define deafness.
2. What is olfaction?
3. What are the sense organs?
4. What are the olfactory organs?
5. Which part of the human ear is responsible for maintaining the body balance?

TRUE/FALSE

1. We have four taste zones.
   A. True   B. False
2. The outer layer of the skin is dermis.
   A. True   B. False
3. The epidermis is the thinnest on your lips.
   A. True   B. False
4. Your nose is made of bones.
   A. True   B. False

Chapter 10: Sense Organs

5. Eyes are the most sensitive and complex sense organ of the body.
   A. True   B. False

MULTIPLE CHOICE QUESTIONS

1. Which organs involve in the sensation of the body?
   a. Organ system   b. Muscular system
   c. Nervous tissue   d. Sensory organs
2. What is known as the "window of the brain"?
   a. Sensory organs   b. Cranial nerves
   c. Eyes   d. Ganglia
3. What helps in maintaining the shape of the eye?
   a. Neuroglia   b. Aqueous humor
   c. Vitreous humor   d. Perikaryon
4. Which organ builds sense of balance?
   a. Respiratory system   b. Auditory system
   c. Vestibular system   d. Digestive system
5. The outer protective covering of human body is known as:
   a. Receptor   b. Skin
   c. Layer   d. Sensory cell
6. The image cast on our retinas is:
   a. Three-dimensional   b. Two-dimensional
   c. Four-dimensional   d. Three-dimensional
7. Taste cells on our tongue that receive the stimulation of taste are known as:
   a. Taste buds   b. Cotton buds
   c. Receptors   d. Tube
8. The human nervous system is capable of a wide range of functions. What is the basic unit of the nervous system?
   a. Glial cell   b. Meninges
   c. Neuron   d. Cerebrospinal fluid
9. The neuron cell is made up of which of the following parts?
   a. Axon   b. Dendrite
   c. Nucleus   d. All of the above

ANSWERS KEY

1. d   2. a   3. c   4. c   5. b
6. b   7. a   8. c   9. d

CHAPTER 11

Endocrine System

INTRODUCTION

The endocrine system is a system responsible for the control of the body's various functions. It is composed of ductless glands that directly secrete hormones into the bloodstream. The chemical messenger secreted by endocrine glands is hormones. The hormones are combined with the circulation of the blood directly and function on another organ or target or tissue. Two systems, one is the central nervous system and the other is the endocrine system, specifically hormones, control everything within the body **(Fig. 11.1)**.

Different endocrine glands are:
- Pituitary gland
- Thyroid gland
- Parathyroid gland
- Adrenal gland
- Pineal gland
- Ovaries in female
- Testes in the male

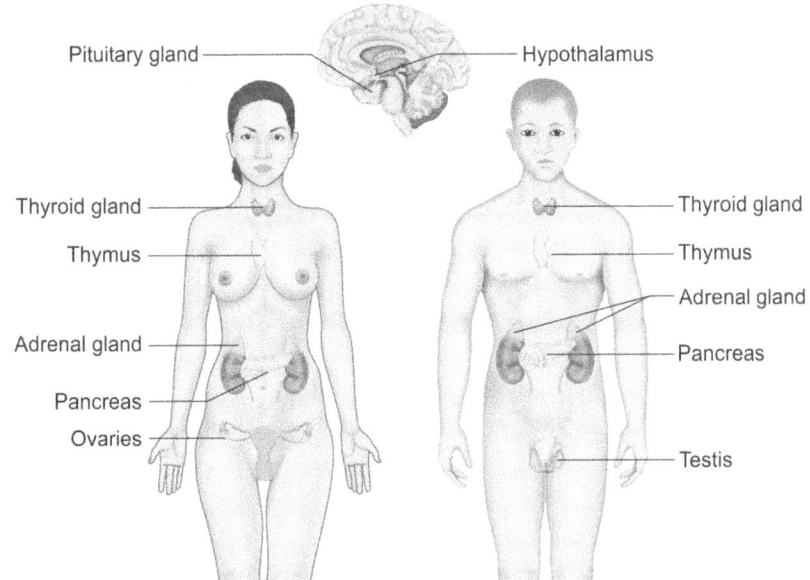

Fig. 11.1: Endocrine system.

Chapter 11: Endocrine System

Functions of endocrine system are:
- To synthesize hormones that control growth and development, metabolism, emotions, organs, and reproduction in an individual.
- To release certain hormones into the bloodstream to allow them to easily enter any other part of the body.

Location of the glands:
Together several glands create the endocrine system:
- The hypothalamus, pituitary gland, and pineal gland are located in the brain.
- The thyroid and parathyroid glands are in the neck region.
- The thymus is present in between lungs
- The adrenals are present on kidneys, and the pancreas behind the stomach.
- Ovaries or testes are situated in the pelvic region.

PITUITARY GLAND

Pituitary gland is the master gland because it secretes hormones that control other endocrine glands. Pituitary gland is governed by hypothalamus and hypothalamus connects the endocrine system to the nervous system. Hypothalamus releases the releasing hormone to direct the pituitary gland to start or stop hormone production (**Fig. 11.2**).

Hormones secreted by the anterior pituitary are:
- **Growth hormone:** It is important for an individual's body to grow and develop. Somatotrophs are synthesized and their release is stimulated by the hypothalamus. As the name suggests the growth hormone stimulates the development of skeleton, tissues and organs, etc.

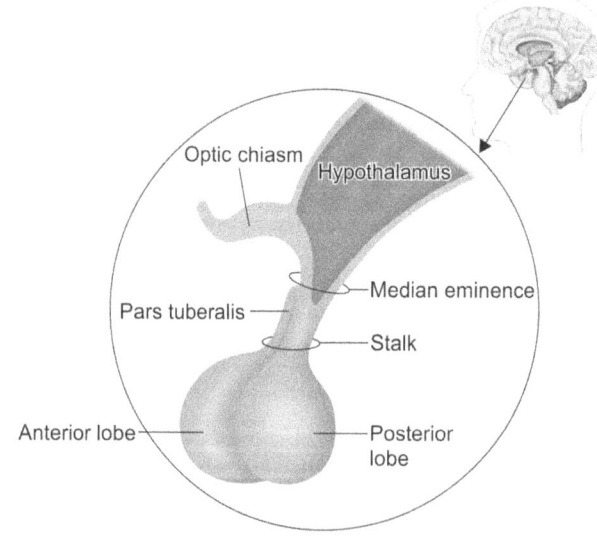

Fig. 11.2: Pituitary gland.

- **Thyrotrophic hormone (TSH):** Thyroid stimulating hormone is stimulated by TRH (thyroid releasing hormone), which is secreted by hypothalamus. The thyroid gland secretes thyroxine (T4) and triiodothyronine (T3) hormones.
- **Adrenocorticotropic hormone (ACTH):** This stimulates the adrenal cortex to synthesize its hormones.
- **Prolactin:** Prolactin hormone acts on breasts after parturition. Prolactin is involved in the maintenance of lactation along with insulin, estrogens, corticosteroids, and thyroxin.
- **Gonadotrophic hormones:** The two gonadotropic hormones in both males and females that are secreted from the anterior pituitary include follicle stimulating hormone (FSH) and luteinizing hormone (LH).
    - In females, FSH stimulates the ovarian follicle production and LH promotes the ovulation.
    - In males, FSH stimulates the development of spermatozoa and LH stimulates interstitial cells for testosterone hormone secretion.
- **Oxytocin:** At the time of birth, oxytocin facilitates the contraction of uterine muscle. It also helps in milk ejection.
- **Antidiuretic hormone or vasopressin:** Antidiuretic hormone increases tubular reabsorption (mainly water absorption) in the kidney. Therefore, it is responsible for rising blood pressure and reducing urine production.

THYROID GLAND

Thyroid gland is located in the thyroid cartilage area of the neck. It has a rich supply of blood. There are two lobes in the thyroid gland, one on either side of the trachea. The two lobes are connected by isthmus (**Fig. 11.3**).

The synthesis of these hormones takes place in four steps:
1. The iodide is removed from the plasma and concentrated in the thyroid gland.
2. Oxidized iodide to iodine
3. Iodide combines with tyrosine and monoiodotyrosine (MIT) and diiodotyrosine (DIT).
4. The two DIT molecules are bound together to form tetraiodothyronine (thyroxine)

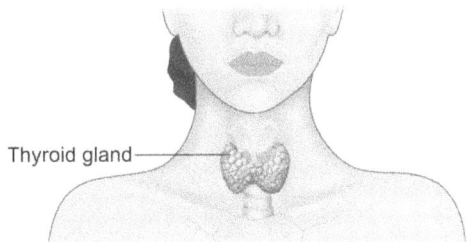

Fig. 11.3: Thyroid gland.

The secretion of thyroid hormone is controlled by TSH, which is secreted from anterior pituitary.

Functions of thyroid gland are:
- It increase the basal metabolic rate of the body
- It increases the heat production in the tissues
- It increases the oxygen consumption and utilization of glucose.
- It helps in storage of the iodine.
- It increases the rate of synthesis of cholesterol and protein, which affects the growth of the individual.

PARATHYROID GLAND

The parathyroid glands are situated behind the thyroid. Parathyroid gland secretes the parathyroid hormone which maintains the levels of calcium and phosphorus in blood within normal limits (**Fig. 11.4**).

ADRENAL OR SUPRARENAL GLANDS

Adrenal glands are two in number and situated on the upper side of the kidney (**Fig. 11.5**).

Adrenal gland can be divided into two parts:
1. An inner medulla
2. An outer cortex

Adrenal Cortex

It secretes three types of hormones mineralocorticoids, glucocorticoids, and sex steroids.

Glucocorticoids

It constitutes cortisol (hydrocortisone), corticosterone, and cortisone. Its secretion is stimulated by stress and adrenocorticotrophic hormone (ACTH). The important functions are:
- Regulation of carbohydrate metabolism
- It helps in formation and storage of glycogen

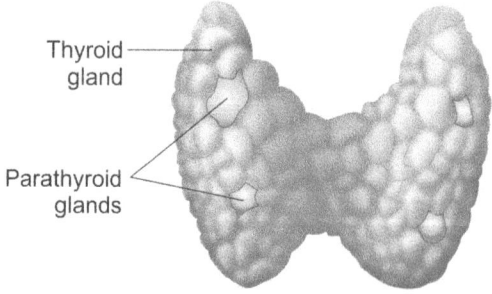

Fig. 11.4: Parathyroid gland.

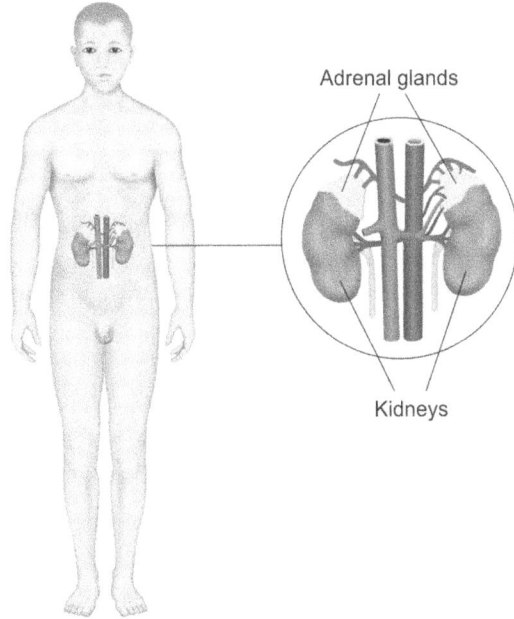

Fig. 11.5: Adrenal gland.

- It helps in raising the blood glucose level by doing gluconeogenesis from protein.
- Reabsorption of sodium and water from renal tubules.
- It helps in distribution of fats.
- It plays an important role in anti-inflammatory and anti-allergic effects.

Mineralocorticoids (Aldosterone)

Aldosterone and deoxycorticosterone are the main mineralocorticoids. By promoting the reabsorption of sodium by renal tubules, it plays an important role in maintaining electrolyte and water balance in the body.

When the amount of reabsorbed sodium is increased, the excretion of potassium is decreased.

Sex Steroids

The hormones that affect growth and sex development in individuals are androgens (male) and estrogen (females).

Adrenal Medulla

The adrenal medulla consists of chromaffin cells, which produce adrenaline and noradrenaline hormones.

Adrenaline comprises about 80% of the total secretion of the gland. Noradrenaline is a chemical transmitter of sympathetic nervous system and responsible for flight, fright and fight response during emergency.

Chapter 11: Endocrine System

Following are the functions of adrenaline and noradrenaline hormone.
- Constriction of the blood vessels
- Dilation of the pupils, bronchioles and blood vessels of muscle
- Increase rate of the heart and force of constriction
- Slowdown the digestion rate

PANCREAS

The pancreas is a part of both your digestive and endocrine systems. The pancreas are present in front of the abdominal aorta and lumbar vertebrae (Fig. 11.6).

The islets of Langerhans are endocrine glands of pancreas. In includes alpha cells (20%), beta cells (70%), delta cells (5%), and F-cells (5%) are four kinds of endocrine cells.

Alpha Cells of Islets of Langerhans

It secretes glucagon. Glucagon raises the amount of blood glucose by mobilizing liver glycogen.

Beta Cells of Islets of Langerhans

It secretes insulin. Insulin helps to reduce blood glucose levels. It enhances glycogen production, improves muscle glucose uptake and facilitates the conversion of glucose into fat into adipose tissue. It also prevents gluconeogenesis (synthesis of glucose).

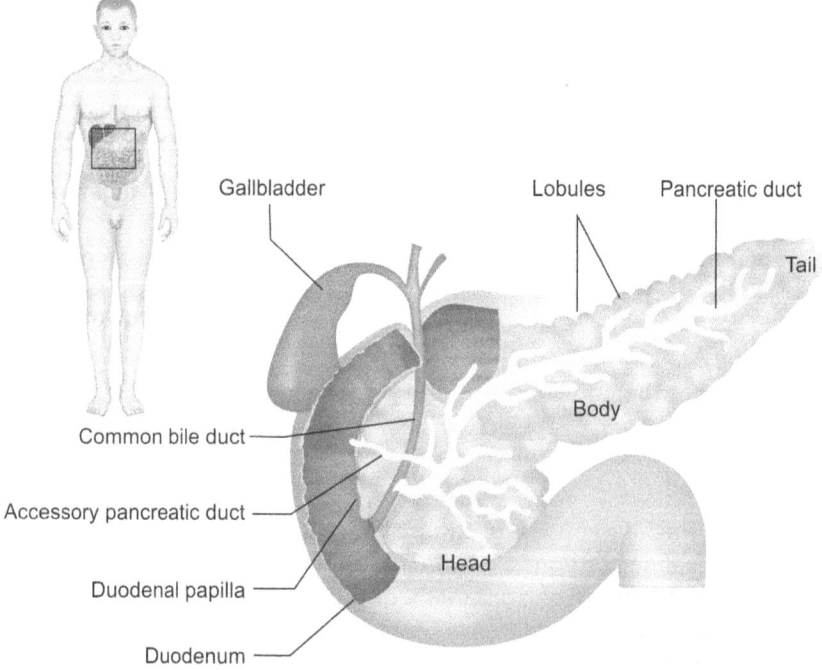

Fig. 11.6: Pancreas.

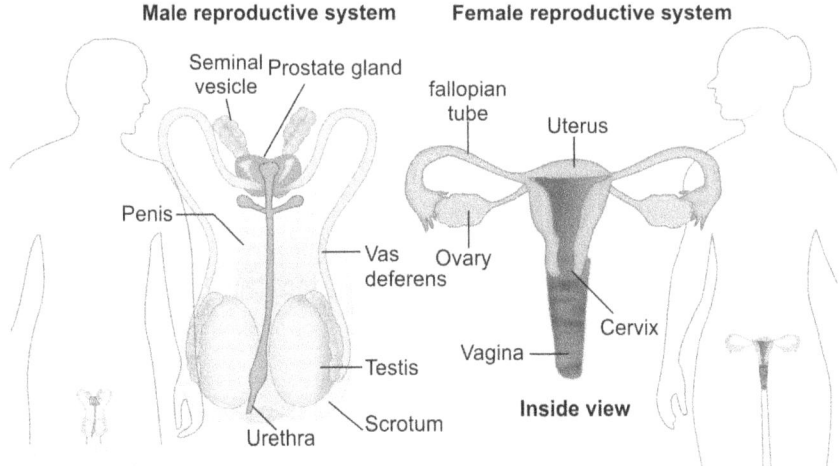

Fig. 11.7: Ovaries and testes.

OVARIES AND TESTES (GONADS)

The sex glands are ovaries and testes. Ovaries in females produce estrogen and progesterone. Testes in males secrete testosterone (**Fig. 11.7**).

Estrogen: It helps to control the menstrual cycle and establishes secondary sexual characteristics of women. The secretion is stimulated by follicle stimulating hormone.

Progesterone: It helps in maturation and development of uterus and breast in females.

Androgens: The most important androgen is testosterone. It helps in growth and development of the male reproductive system, muscle enlargement, and growth of body hair.

THYMUS

Thymus is situated on trachea. It secretes four hormones, namely, thymosin, thymic factor, thymic humoral factor (THF), and thymopoietin.

It helps in production of lymphocytes, which help in proliferation and maturation of T-lymphocytes (**Fig. 11.8**).

PINEAL GLAND

Pineal gland is the small gland, which is located in brain. Pineal gland produces melatonin, which maintain circadian rhythm and sleep cycle.

ENDOCRINE SYSTEM DISORDERS

Acromegaly

Acromegaly is a hormonal disorder, which is characterized by enlarged bones of hands, feet, and face due to increased production of growth hormone. It usually starts at an early age.

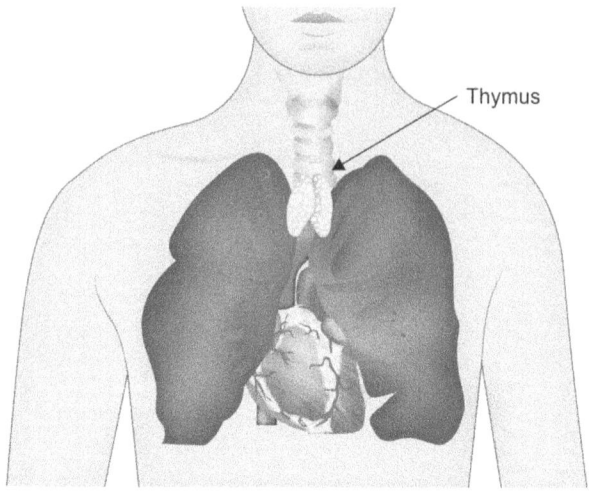

Fig. 11.8: Thymus gland.

Adrenal Insufficiency

In this adrenal gland does not make enough of certain hormones, like cortisol, which controls stress.

Cushing's Disease

In this, the body makes too much cortisol. Patients can gain weight, get stretch marks, bruises, weakened muscles and bones and possibly develop a hump on your upper back **(Fig. 11.9)**.

Hyperthyroidism

Thyroid gland produces more hormones than its requirement. It makes body system runs fast and one might feel nervous, lose weight, and have a rapid heartbeat or trouble in sleeping.

Hypothyroidism

When your body does not make enough thyroid hormone, the system slows down. Patients might feel tired, gain weight, have a slow heartbeat, and have joint and muscle pains.

Hypopituitarism

In this, pituitary gland does not make enough of certain hormones.

Polycystic Ovary Syndrome

An imbalance of reproductive hormones, which causes ovaries either not make an egg or not release it during ovulation. This can cause disturbance in periods. It causes acne and makes hair to grow on your face or chin.

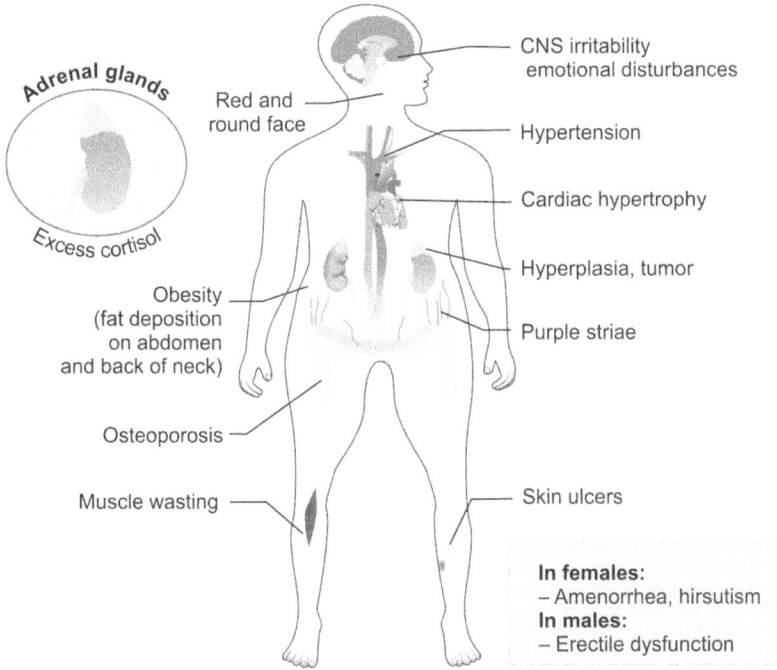

Fig. 11.9: Cushing syndrome.

Gigantism

Gigantism occurs when growth hormone is overproduced by the pituitary gland and the bones and parts of the body of a child start to develop abnormally rapidly. Contrarily, if too little growth hormone is developed by the gland, the child will stop increasing in height.

Endocrine Tumors

Endocrine gland tumors are normally noncancerous. They do not spread to other components of the body. Medicinal products or surgery can treat hyperfunctional endocrine tumors.

Grave's Disease

Grave's disease is the most common form of hyperthyroidism. It occurs when immune system does not recognize body cells and mistakenly attacks the thyroid gland. It causes it to overproduce the hormone thyroxine.

Hypoglycemia

Hypoglycemia is a condition of low blood sugar, occurs when blood glucose level drops too low to provide enough energy for the body's activities. Symptoms are unconsciousness or seizures due to low blood sugar.

Hypogonadism

When a man's testes fail to produce sufficient quantities of testosterone and/or sperm quality is impaired.

Diabetes

Diabetes is a disease in which blood glucose levels are abnormal. The body of a person with diabetes either does not make enough insulin or it is resistant to utilize insulin in the body.

SUMMARY

- The endocrine system is a system that is responsible for the regulation of different functions of the body.
- The endocrine system consists of glands or ductless glands that secrete hormones directly to the bloodstream.
- Hormones are the chemical messenger secreted by endocrine glands.
- Different endocrine glands are (**Table 11.1**):
  - Pituitary gland
  - Thyroid gland
  - Parathyroid gland
  - Adrenal gland
  - Pineal gland
  - Ovaries in female
  - Testes in the male
- Location of the glands:
  - The hypothalamus, pituitary gland, and pineal gland are located in the brain.
  - The thyroid and parathyroid glands are in the neck region.
  - The thymus is present in between lungs.
  - The adrenals are present on kidneys, and the pancreas behind the stomach.
  - Ovaries or testes are situated in the pelvic region.
- Pituitary gland known as master gland because it secretes hormones that control other endocrine glands. Hormones secreted by the anterior pituitary are growth hormone, thyrotrophic hormone (TSH), adrenocorticotropic hormone (ACTH), prolactin, gonadotrophic hormones, oxytocin, antidiuretic hormone or vasopressin.
- **Thyroid gland:** It is situated in the neck region on the thyroid cartilage. It increases the basal metabolic rate of the body; it increases the heat production in the tissues, oxygen consumption and utilization of glucose, helps in storage of the Iodine.
- **Parathyroid:** This gland controls the levels of calcium and phosphorus.
- **Adrenal or suprarenal glands:** It secretes three types of hormones mineralo-corticoids, glucocorticoids, and sex steroid.
- **Pancreas:** This organ is part of both your digestive and endocrine systems. The islets of Langerhans are islets in the pancreatic tissue which are endocrine glands. It secretes Glucagon. Glucagon increases blood glucose level by mobilizing glycogen from liver. It secretes insulin, which helps in decreasing the level of glucose in the blood.
- **Ovaries and testes (gonads):** Ovaries in females produce estrogen and progesterone. Testes in males secrete testosterone.
- **Thymus:** It is situated on trachea. It helps in the production of T-lymphocytes.

TABLE 11.1: Different endocrine glands.

Gland	Hormone	Target tissue	Response
Pituitary gland anterior	Growth hormone	Body tissues	Stimulates growth of bone and tissue, increases gene expression, breakdown of lipids, release of fatty acids from the cells increases blood glucose level
	Thyroid stimulating hormone	Thyroid gland	Stimulate thyroid gland to produce thyroid hormones (thyroxine and triiodothyronine)
	Adrenocorticotrophic hormone	Adrenal cortex	Stimulate adrenal gland to produce several hormones, increases secretion of glucocorticoid hormones such as cortisol
	Luteinizing hormone	Ovaries in females and testes in males	Stimulate sexual function and production of the sex steroids, ovulation and progesterone production in females or testosterone synthesis and support for sperm cell production in males
	Follicle stimulating hormone	Follicle in ovaries in females, testes in males	Promotes follicle maturation and estrogen secretion in ovaries, promotes sperm cell production in testis
	Melanocyte stimulating hormone	Melanocyte in skin	Increases melanin production in melanocyte to make skin darker
Pituitary gland posterior	Antidiuretic hormone	Kidney	Conserves water, constricts blood vessels
	Oxytocin	Uterus	Increases uterine contraction
		Mammary glands	Milk ejection
Thyroid gland	Thyroxine and triiodothyronine hormones	Most cells of body	Increases metabolic rate, essential for normal process of growth and maturation.
	Calcitonin	Bones	Decreases the rate of bone breakdown, reduces calcium level in blood after large meal

Contd...

Contd...

Gland	Hormone	Target tissue	Response
Parathyroid gland	Parathyroid hormone	Bones and kidney	Increases the rate of bone breakdown by osteoclasts, increases vitamin D synthesis, essential for maintenance of normal calcium level in blood
Adrenal medulla	Epinephrine Nor epinephrine	Heart, blood vessels, liver, fat cells	Increases cardiac output, increases blood flow to skeletal muscles and heart, increases release of glucose and fatty acids into blood
Adrenal cortex	Mineral corticosteroids	Kidney, intestine and sweat glands	Increases the rate of sodium transport into body, increases the rate of potassium excretion, favor water retention
	Glucocorticoids	Liver, fat, skeletal muscle, immune tissues	Increases fat and protein breakdown, increases gluconeogenesis, inhibit inflammation and immune response
	Androgens	Most tissues	Increases libido in females, insignificant in males, growth of pubic and axillary hair
Pancreas	Insulin Glucagon	Liver, skeletal muscle, and adipose tissues	Regulate carbohydrate metabolism by secreting Insulin and glucagon
Gonads	Ovaries (estrogen)	Lower abdomen	Controls the regulation of the female reproductive system, including menstrual cycle and pregnancy
	Testes (testosterone)	Scrotum	Responsible for the development of male sex characteristics during puberty, while also promoting muscle growth
Thymus	Thymosin	Behind the sternum (breastbone) but in front of the heart	It stimulates the development of disease-fighting T-cells
Pineal gland	Melatonin	epithalamus	Responsible for important biological rhythms, including the sleep-wake cycle

Chapter 11: Endocrine System

GLOSSARY

1. **Acromegaly:** It is a hormonal disorder where the pituitary gland produces excess amounts of growth hormone.
2. **Adrenal cortex:** The adrenal cortex is the outer portion of the adrenal gland and it produces steroid hormones, which regulate carbohydrate and fat metabolism, and mineralocorticoid hormones, which regulate salt and water balance in the body.
3. **Adrenal glands:** They regulate stress response through the synthesis of hormones, including cortisol and adrenaline.
4. **Adrenaline:** It is a hormone that triggers the body's fight-or-flight response. It is produced in the medulla in the adrenal glands as well as some of the central nervous system's neurons.
5. **Adrenocorticotropin (ACTH):** Adrenocorticotropin is a hormone produced by the anterior pituitary gland that stimulates the adrenal cortex.
6. **Amenorrhea:** When a woman or adolescent girl is not having menstrual periods.
7. **Androgens:** Hormones that help to develop sex organs in men. They also contribute to sexual function in men and women.
8. **Andropause:** It is a biological change characterized by a gradual decline in androgens experienced by men. Andropause is sometimes described as male menopause.
9. **Calcitonin:** It inhibits cells that break down bone and helps to regulate the blood's calcium and phosphate levels.
10. **Cortisol:** It is produced by the adrenal gland. It is involved in the stress response and increases blood pressure and blood sugar levels.
11. **Endocrinologist:** Specially trained physicians who diagnose diseases related to the glands.
12. **Erythropoietin:** It is a hormone directly connected to red blood cell production and maintenance.
13. **Estradiol:** Female sex hormone produced mainly by the ovaries. It is responsible for growth of breast tissue, maturation of long bones, and development of the secondary sexual characteristics.
14. **Estrogen:** Group of steroid compounds that are the primary female sex hormones. They promote the development of female secondary sex characteristics and control aspects of regulating the menstrual cycle.
15. **Glands:** They produce and secrete hormones that the body uses for a wide range of functions.
16. **Glucagon:** Glucagon is a hormone that works with other hormones and bodily functions to control glucose levels in the blood.
17. **Gonads:** A gonad is an organ that produces sperm and egg cells known as gametes. The gonads in males are the testes, and the gonads in females are the ovaries.
18. **Hormones:** Hormones are chemical messengers that travel in the bloodstream to tissues.
19. **Hypothalamus:** This is an area of the brain that regulates vital autonomic centers and produces hormones that control thirst, hunger, body temperature, sleep, moods, sex drive, and the release of hormones from various glands, primarily the pituitary gland.
20. **Insulin:** It is a protein pancreatic hormone involved in the metabolism of carbohydrates and the regulation of glucose levels in the blood. Diabetes occurs when the body does not produce enough insulin or use the hormone effectively.

Chapter 11: Endocrine System

LONG ANSWER TYPE QUESTIONS

1. What are endocrine glands?
2. Name the endocrine gland of the body and write the functions.
3. List the hormones secreted by anterior pituitary and posterior pituitary gland and list functions of the thyroid gland.

SHORT ANSWER TYPE QUESTIONS

1. Islets of Langerhans of pancreas.
2. Antidiuretic hormone.
3. Pineal gland.
4. Male and female sex hormones.

MULTIPLE CHOICE QUESTIONS

1. Glands are small organs located throughout body that secretes:
   - a. Plasma
   - b. Hormones
   - c. Enzymes
   - d. Bile
2. Which of the following is not part of the endocrine system?
   - a. Thyroid
   - b. Adrenals
   - c. Appendix
   - d. Pituitary
3. This gland is sometimes called the master gland:
   - a. Pituitary
   - b. Adrenal
   - c. Pineal
   - d. Hypothalamus
4. What hormone does the pancreas make?
   - a. Insulin
   - b. Adrenaline
   - c. Growth hormones
   - d. Sugar
5. Which of the following is NOT an endocrine gland?
   - a. Hypothalamus
   - b. Pituitary
   - c. Parathyroid
   - d. Pancreas

ANSWERS KEY

1. b   2. c   3. a   4. a   5. a

Chapter 11: Endocrine System

ATLAS

Identify and label the diagrams.

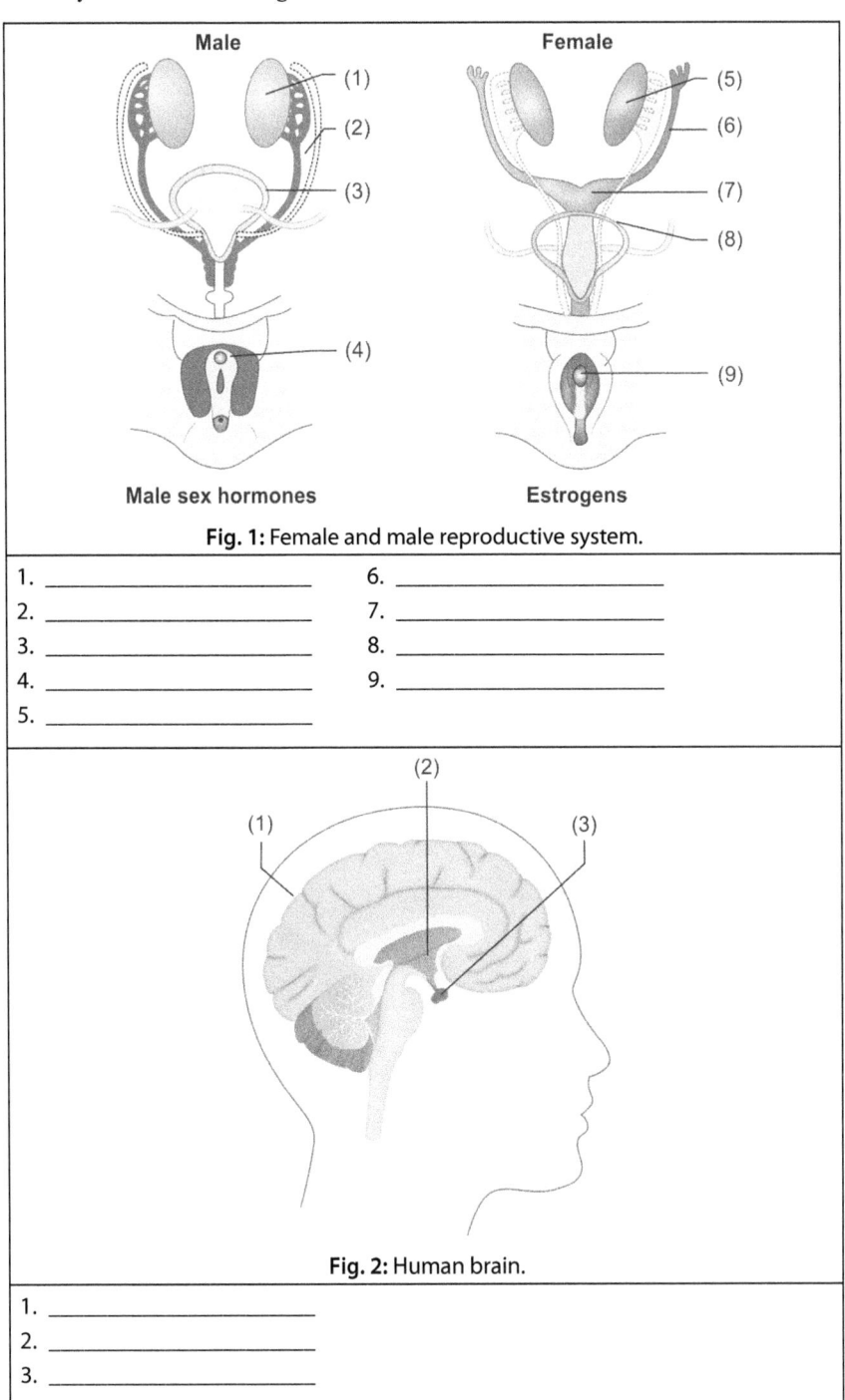

Fig. 1: Female and male reproductive system.

1. _____
2. _____
3. _____
4. _____
5. _____
6. _____
7. _____
8. _____
9. _____

Fig. 2: Human brain.

1. _____
2. _____
3. _____

Chapter 11: Endocrine System

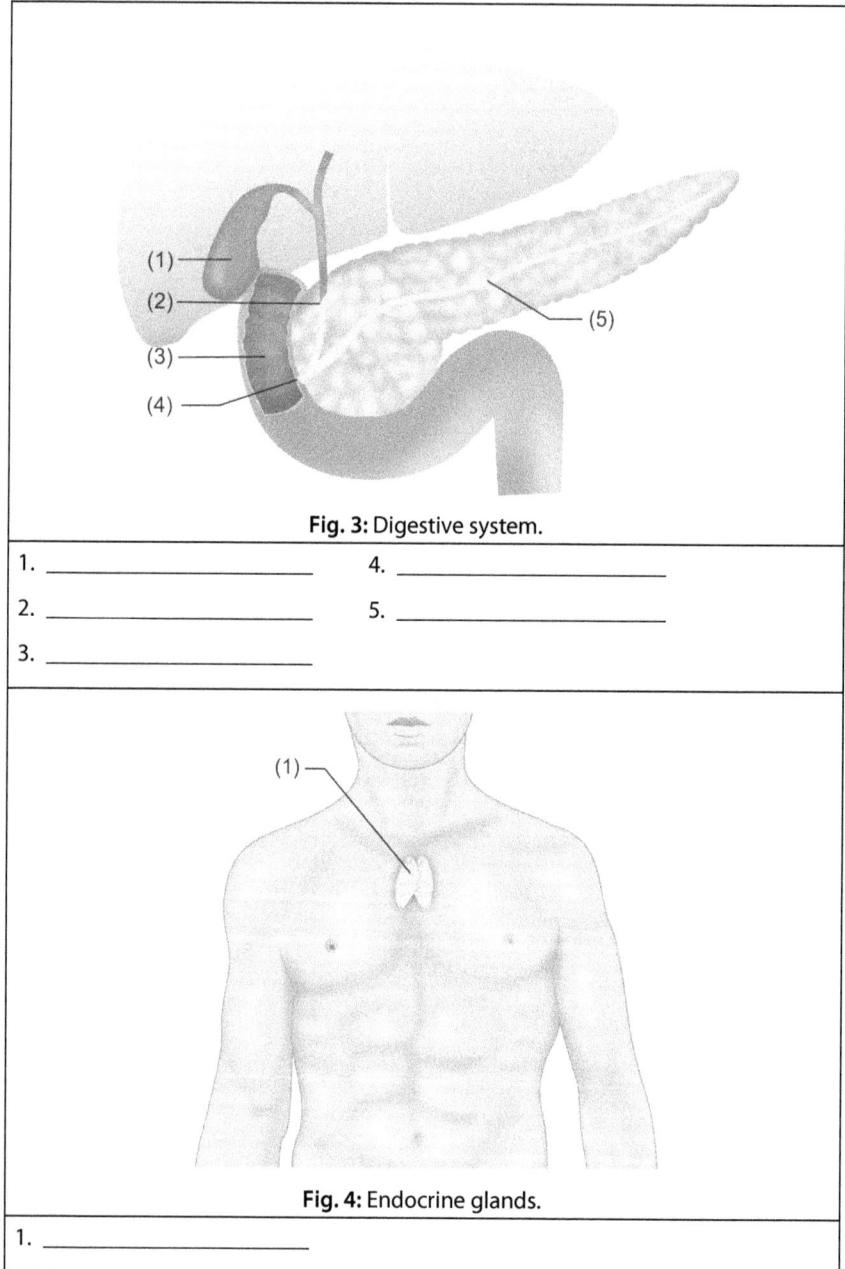

Fig. 3: Digestive system.

1. _____
2. _____
3. _____
4. _____
5. _____

Fig. 4: Endocrine glands.

1. _____

Chapter 11: Endocrine System 137

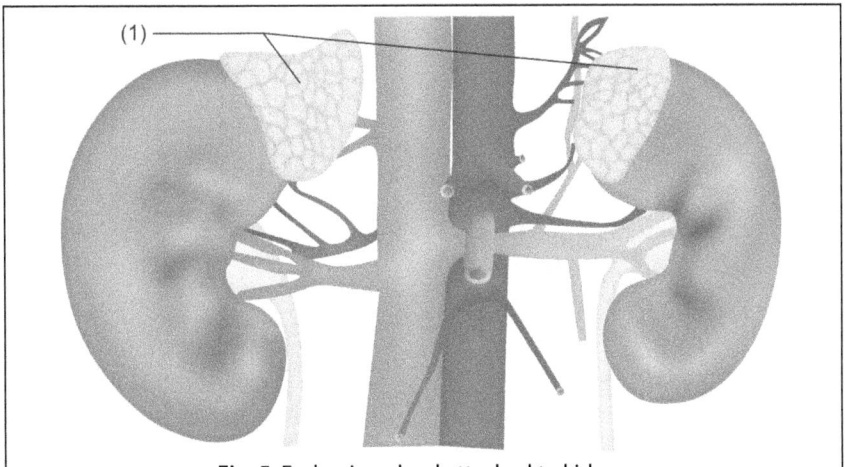

Fig. 5: Endocrine gland attached to kidney.

1. _____

Fig. 6: Endocrine glands of the body.

1. _____ 6. _____
2. _____ 7. _____
3. _____ 8. _____
4. _____ 9. _____
5. _____

CHAPTER 12

Reproductive System

INTRODUCTION

Reproductive system is consists of all the organs that are responsible in producing new off spring. Reproductive system comprises of internal and external organs both in males and females.

The female reproductive organ produces ova through oogenesis and male reproductive organ produces sperms through spermatogenesis. Ova and sperms fuse together to produce offspring.

Function of Male Reproductive System
- To produce male sex hormone.
- To eject the sperm into female reproductive system
- To nurture, produce, and transfer the sperms and protective fluid.

MALE REPRODUCTIVE SYSTEM

The external male genital organs or reproductive organs consist of (**Fig. 12.1**):
- Penis
- Scrotum
- Testes
- Epididymis

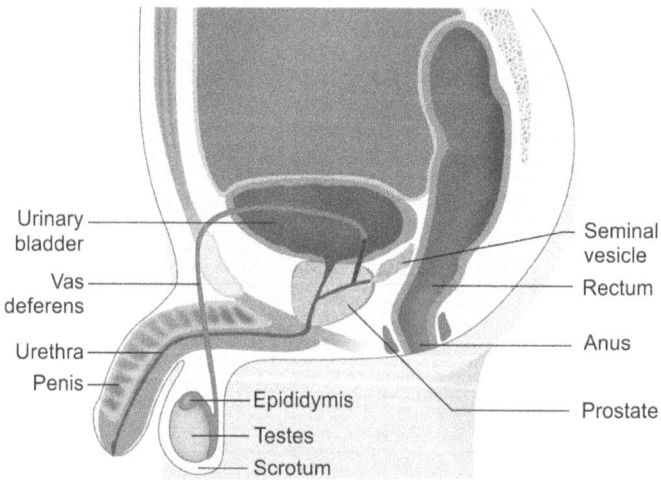

Fig. 12.1: External male genital organs.

The External Male Genital Organs

Penis

- Penis is composed of specialized erectile tissues. It contains the urethra which is a common outlet for both urine and semen.
- The parasympathetic nerve stimulation causes the erection of penis.
- The blood supply for the penis is from the **penile artery**.
- The glans is a sensitive, bulging ridge of tissue. It is located at the distal part of the penis. The skin covering the glans penis is called the **prepuce or foreskin**. The prepuce or foreskin is retractable casing of skin, protects the glans at birth.
- Prepuce or foreskin is the part that is surgically removed during **circumcision**.

Scrotum

- Scrotum is skin-covered pouch over the perineum, which is located at the base of penis.
- The scrotum provides support to the testes and is responsible for regulation of temperature (less temperature than body) of the sperm, which is requisite for the production of sperms.
- It is rugated, muscular, and bilobed structure, which is covered by pubic hair externally.
- To promote the production and viability of the sperm, the scrotum contracts toward the body during a very cold weather and relaxes away from the body during a hot weather.

Testes

- Testes are the primary male reproductive organ. Just before birth testes descend through a canal into an external sac called the scrotum (**Fig. 12.2**).

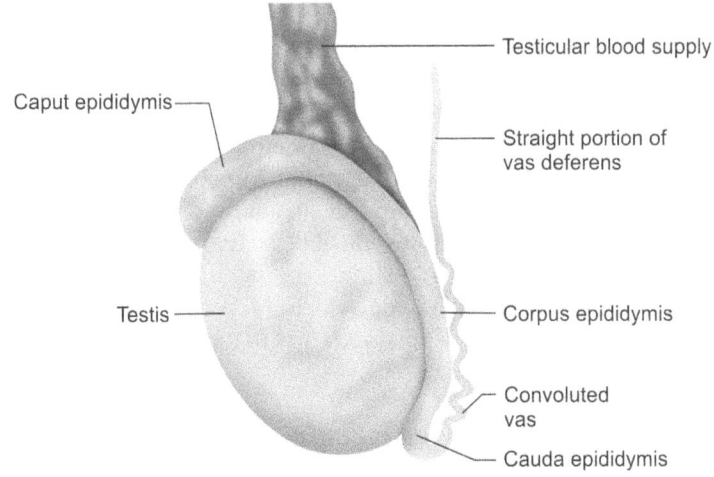

Fig. 12.2: Testes.

- Testes lie into scrotum. Each scrotum has two testes.
- Testes are 2-3 cm wide and covered with tough, fibrous layer of tissue called tunica.
- Testes are composed of various testicles, which also contain Leydig's cells. These Leydig's cells produce testosterone.
- The seminiferous tubules located in testes produce spermatozoa.
- In most men, one testis is slightly lower than the other to prevent trauma and easily sit or do any muscular activity.

Epididymis
- This is a tightly coiled tube, which is responsible for conducting the sperm from the seminiferous tubule to the vas deferens.
- The length of epididymis is approximately 20 feet.
- It also serves the storage of sperms, along with the semen.
- The sperm takes an estimated 12-20 days of travel along the epididymis, and a total of 64 days to reach maturity.

The internal male genital organs or reproductive organs consists of:
- Vas deferens
- Prostate gland
- Ejaculatory duct
- Seminal vesicles
- Urethra in penis

The Internal Male Genital Organs (Fig. 12.3)

Vas Deferens
- The function of the vas deferens is to carry the sperm through the inguinal canal from the epididymis into the abdominal cavity where it will join at the seminal vesicles and the ejaculatory duct.
- It is a hollow tube, which is protected by a thick fibrous coating.
- It is surrounded by arteries and veins.

Prostate Gland
- Prostate gland situated below the urinary bladder.
- The weight of prostate gland is approximately 8 g, which progressively increases in size by the age of 50 years approximately 40 g.
- The milky fluid, which makes around 30% of the semen, is produced by prostate gland. Therefore, it is responsible to give milky appearance to the semen.
- It also consists of clotting enzyme, which thickens the semen inside the vagina, so that semen can be retained close to the cervix.

Seminal Vesicles
- These are two convoluted pouches lie in the lower portion of the posterior surface of the bladder.

Chapter 12: Reproductive System

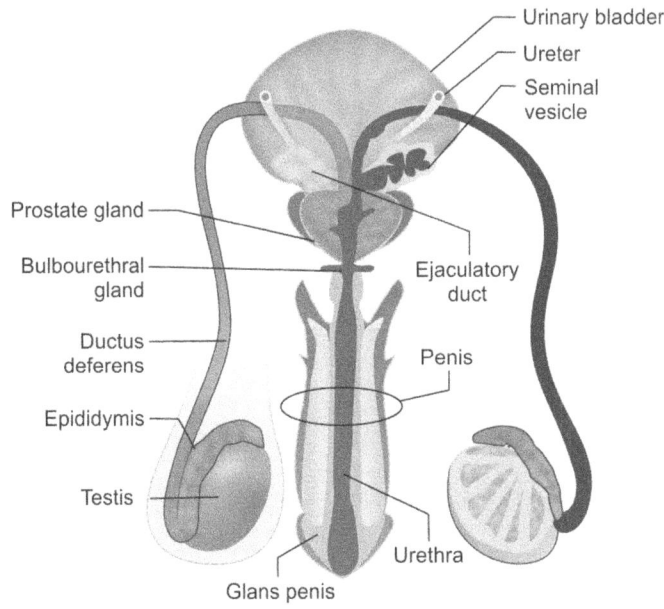

Fig. 12.3: Internal male genital organs.

- The seminal vesicles secrete a viscous liquid. The viscous fluid is alkaline in pH.
- The seminal vesicle fluid has high protein, sugar, and prostaglandin content, which makes the sperm motile.

Ejaculatory Ducts
The ejaculatory ducts pass through the prostate gland to join the seminal vesicles and the urethra.

Urethra
- Urethra passes through the prostate gland toward the glans penis.
- Urethra is a hollow tube starting from the base of the bladder.
- It is lined with mucous membrane.
- It has a length of approximately 8 inches or 18–20 cm

FEMALE REPRODUCTIVE SYSTEM
- The female reproductive system is composed of internal and external genital organs.
- The function of female reproductive system is to produce ova or oocytes, which is required for reproduction.
- The female reproductive system menstruates, if fertilization or implantation does not occur.

Chapter 12: Reproductive System

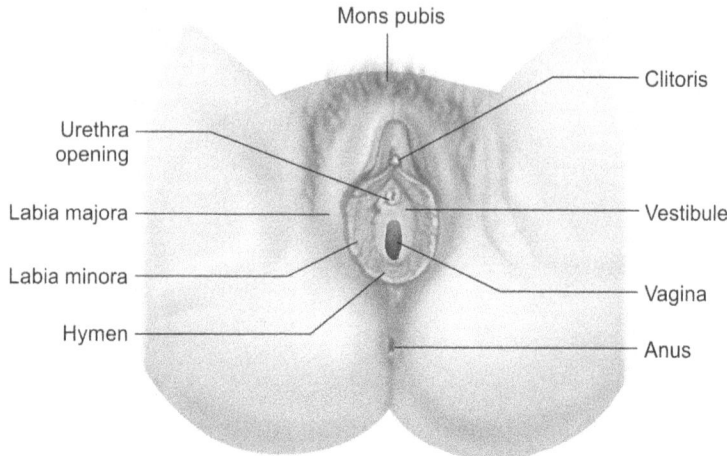

Fig. 12.4: External female reproductive organs.

External Female Reproductive Organ
- Mons pubis
- Labia majora
- Labia Minora
- Clitoris
- Perineum (**Fig. 12.4**)

Mons Pubis
- Mons pubis is rounded, soft fullness of subcutaneous fatty tissue, and it is prominent over the symphysis pubis.
- It forms the external reproductive organ.
- Mons pubis is surrounded by the varying degree of pubic hair.

Labia Majora
- Two rounded, fleshy tissue folds that extend from the mons pubis to the perineum are called as labia majora.
- It protects the labia minora, urinary meatus and vaginal introitus.
- It is coated in pubic hair that provides extra protection from harmful bacteria that can penetrate the structure.

Labia Minora
- The labia minora lies inside the labia majora
- Usually, the lateral and anterior aspects are pigmented.
- The inner surfaces are similar to the pink and moist vaginal mucosa.
- They are high in vascularity.
- The internal surface consists of a mucous membrane and the skin is the external surface. Contains sebaceous glands in the area.

Clitoris
- The term clitoris comes from a Greek word meaning key.
- It is an erectile organ, which can be compared with male penis.
- It is very vascular which has receptors that are highly sensitive to temperature, touch, and pressure.

Perineum
- Perineum is formed by the most posterior part of the external female reproductive organ.
- It extends from fourchette anteriorly to the anus posteriorly.
- It is composed of fibrous and muscular tissues that provide support to the pelvic structures

The functions of the female reproductive system are:
- Ova formation
- Spermatozoa reception
- It provides suitable environment for fertilization and fetal growth.
- It forms birth canal and facilitate in labor and parturition (childbirth)
- Lactation, the processing of breast milk, which in its early life provides full nourishment for the baby.

Internal Female Reproductive Organ (Fig. 12.5)
- Vagina
- Uterus
- Fallopian tubes/uterine tube
- Ovaries
- Cervix

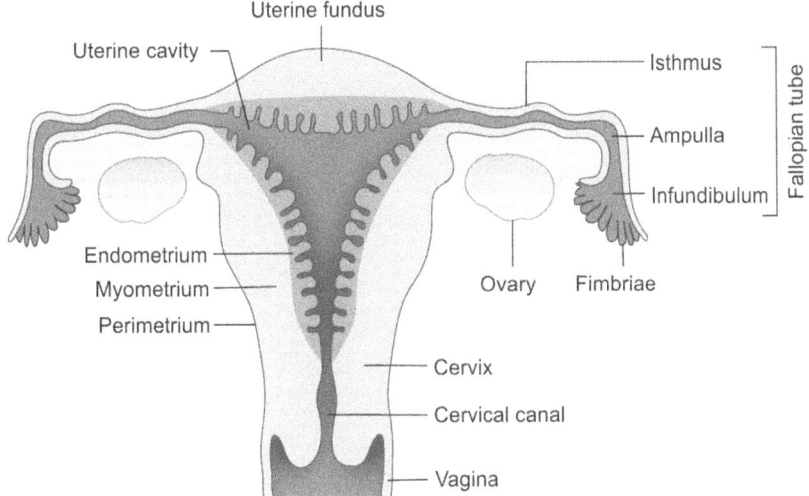

Fig. 12.5: Internal female reproductive organs.

Vagina

- It is an elastic fibro muscular tube roughly 8–10 cm long.
- Lying between the anterior bladder and the posterior rectum. The vagina connects the vestibule below and with the uterus above.
- There are numerous folds, or rugae and muscle sheet, on the vaginal lining. During child birth, these folds cause the vagina to spread significantly.

Uterus

- Uterus is situated in the lower pelvis, which is located anterior to rectum and posterior to bladder.
- The uterus is measured 5–7 cm long and 5 cm wide.
- For nonpregnant mothers, the weight is about 60 g and in pregnant state the weight of uterus is 900 g approximately.
- The purpose of uterus is to accept the ovum from the Fallopian tube
- It provides a place for implantation.
- It also provides nutrition and protection for the growing fetus.
- It is divided into three—the body, the isthmus, and the cervix and fundus (**Fig. 12.6**).

Fallopian Tubes/Uterine Tube

- Fallopian tubes are also known as uterine tubes that connect ovaries to uterus.
- The fallopian tubes serve as the pathway for ovum toward the uterus.
- It is a hollow tube divided into four parts: the interstitial, the isthmus, the ampulla, and the infundibulum.
- **Fertilization occurs in the ampulla.**
- The fallopian tube has small hairs (finger-like projection) called the **fimbria** that propel the ovum into the fallopian tube.

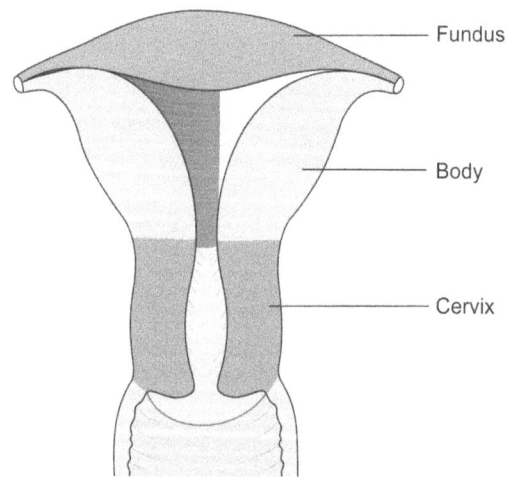

Fig. 12.6: Parts of uterus.

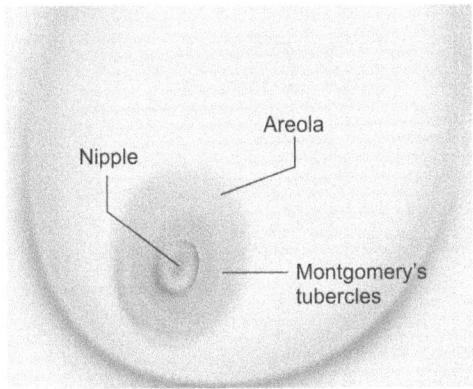

Fig. 12.7: Breast.

Ovaries

- The ovaries create, mature, and discharge the egg cells or ova for its function.
- Ovarian function is meant to mature and retain secondary sex characteristics in women.

Cervix

- It is the lower narrow end of the uterus that forms a canal between uterus and vagina.
- Cervix gets dilated during labor.

Accessory Organ of Female Reproductive System

Breast

- The breast or mammary glands are female accessory glands.
- Breast also appears in the male but only in rudimentary form.
- There are about 20 lobes in each breast, which has structures called lobules, where milk is produced **(Fig. 12.7)**.

MENSTRUAL CYCLE

- Females of reproductive age (beginning anywhere from 11 to 16 years of age) experience hormonal activity cycles, which repeat at intervals of about 1 month. Menstrual means "monthly" and the term menstrual cycle is therefore used **(Fig. 12.8)**.
- The term menstruation refers to the uterine lining's frequent shedding.
- The normal menstrual cycle takes about 28 days and takes place in stages: the follicular process (development of the egg), the ovulatory phase (release of the egg), and the luteal phase (decrease of hormone levels, if the egg is not fertilized).
- There are four major hormones (chemicals that stimulate or regulate the activity of cells or organs) involved in the menstrual cycle: follicle-stimulating hormone, luteinizing hormone, estrogen, and progesterone.

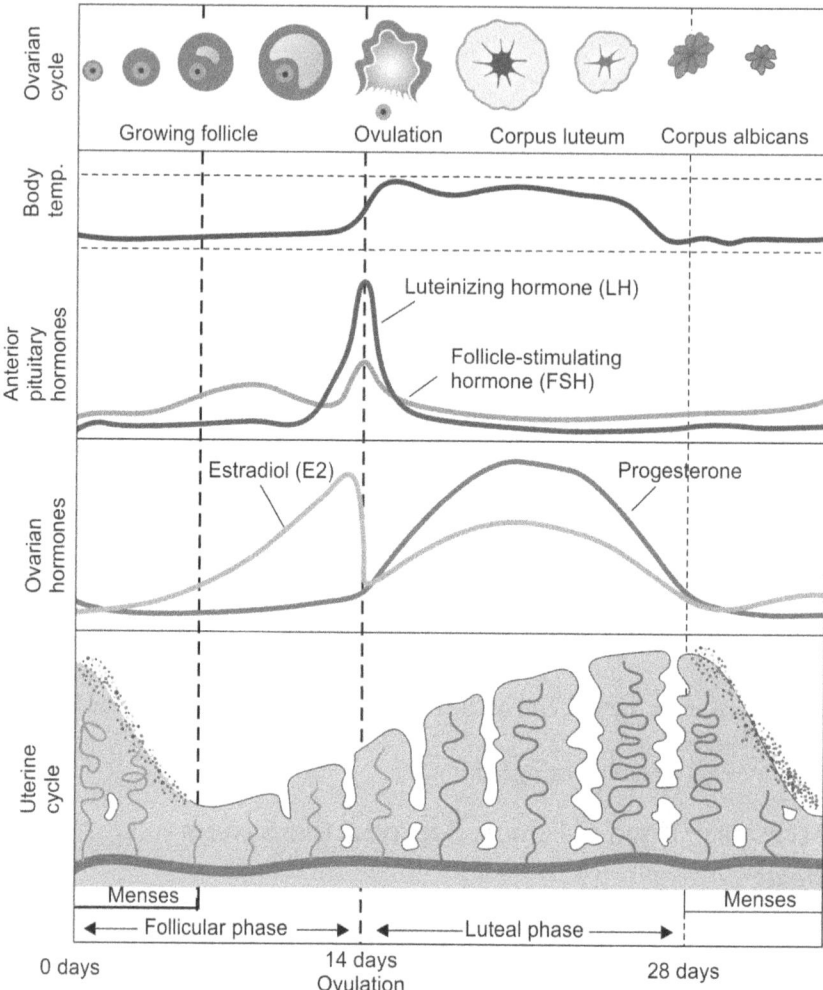

Fig. 12.8: Menstrual cycle.

Follicular Phase

This phase starts on the first day of period. During the follicular phase of the menstrual cycle, the following events occur:
* Two hormones are released from the brain, the follicle stimulating hormone (FSH) and luteinizing hormone (LH), and pass to the ovaries via the blood.
* The hormones promote the development of around 15–20 eggs in the ovaries, each in a follicle called its own "shell". Such hormones (FSH and LH) also allow the development of the female hormone estrogen to increase.
* As estrogen levels rise, like a switch, it turns off the production of FSH. This careful balance of hormones allows the body to limit the number of follicles that will prepare eggs to be released.

- As the follicular phase progresses, one follicle in one ovary becomes dominant and continues to mature. This dominant follicle suppresses all of the other follicles in the group. As a result, they stop growing and die. The dominant follicle continues to produce estrogen.

Ovulatory Phase

The ovulatory phase, or ovulation, starts about 14 days after the follicular phase started. The ovulatory phase is the midpoint of the menstrual cycle, with the next menstrual period starting about 2 weeks later. During this phase, the following events occur:
- The increase of estrogen from the dominant follicle induces as urge in the amount LH.
- This stimulates the dominant follicle to release the ovary from its egg.
- As the egg is released (a process called ovulation) it is captured by finger-like projections on the end of the fallopian tubes (fimbriae). The fimbriae sweep the egg into the tube.
- Also during this phase, there is an increase in the amount and thickness of mucus produced by the cervix (lower part of the uterus). If a woman were to have intercourse during this time, the thick mucus captures the man's sperm, nourishes it, and helps it to move towards the egg for fertilization.

Luteal Phase

- The luteal phase begins right after ovulation and involves the following processes:
- The empty ovarian follicle develops into a new structure called the corpus luteum once it releases its egg.
- The hormones estrogen and progesterone are secreted by the corpus luteum.
- Progesterone prepares the uterus for the implantation of a fertilized egg.
- The fertilized egg (embryo) will pass through the fallopian tube to implant in the uterus if sex has taken place and the sperm of a man has fertilized the egg (a process called conception). The woman is considered to be pregnant now.
- If the egg is not fertilized, it passes through the uterus. Not needed to support a pregnancy, the lining of the uterus breaks down and sheds, and the next menstrual period begins.

REPRODUCTIVE SYSTEM DISORDERS

- **Uterine fibroids:** They are the noncancerous tumor in women and can anywhere in the uterus they are made up of muscle cell and other tissue cells.
- **Interstitial cystitis:** Inflammation of the bladder causing discomfort and pain in the patient.
- **Cryptorchidism:** Failure of one or both of the testes to descend into the scrotum.

Chapter 12: Reproductive System

- **Epispadias:** An opening in the upper side of the penis.
- **Erectile dysfunction:** Inability of the penis to maintain the erection during intercourse.
- **Cancer of cervix:** The malignant neoplasm arising from cells originating in the cervix.

SUMMARY

- Male reproductive system consists of external and internal organs
- **The external male reproductive organs:**
  - Penis
  - Scrotum
  - Testes
  - Epididymis
- **The internal male reproductive organs:**
  - Vas deferens
  - Prostate gland
  - Ejaculatory duct
  - Seminal vesicles
  - Urethra in penis
- **Female reproductive system consists of external and internal organs.**
- **The external female reproductive organs:**
  - Mons pubis
  - Labia majora
  - Labia minora
  - Clitoris
  - Perineum
- **Internal female reproductive organ:**
  - Vagina
  - Uterus
  - Fallopian tubes
  - Ovaries
- **Accessory organ of female reproductive system:** The breasts or mammary glands are accessory glands of the female reproductive system
- **Menstrual cycle:**
  - The average menstrual cycle takes about 28 days and occurs in phases: the follicular phase (development of the egg), the ovulatory phase (release of the egg), and the luteal phase (hormone levels decrease if the egg is not fertilized).
  - *Follicular phase:* This phase starts on the first day of period
  - *Ovulatory phase:* The ovulatory phase, or ovulation, starts about 14 days after the follicular phase started. The ovulatory phase is the midpoint of the menstrual cycle, with the next menstrual period starting about 2 weeks later
  - *Luteal phase:* The luteal phase begins right after ovulation.

GLOSSARY

1. **Infertility:** The inability to get pregnant or sustain a pregnancy.
2. **Ovary:** Part of the female reproductive system. There are two ovaries, located on either side of the uterus. They contain and produce eggs and hormones.

Chapter 12: Reproductive System

3. **Ovulation:** When an ovary releases an egg into the fallopian tube. The process is called ovulation.
4. **Fertilization:** The process whereby male and female **gametes** (**sperm** and **egg**) unite.
5. **Reproduction:** The natural process among organisms by which new individuals are generated and the species perpetuated.
6. **Gametes** are an organism's reproductive cells. They are also referred to as sex cells. Female **gametes** are called ova or egg cells, and male **gametes** are called sperm.
7. **Semen**, also called seminal fluid, fluid that is emitted from the male reproductive tract and that contains sperm cells, which are capable of fertilizing the female's eggs. **Semen** also contains liquids that combine to form seminal plasma, which helps keep the sperm cells viable.

LONG ANSWER TYPE QUESTION

1. Define menstrual cycle and explain the process of menstruation.

SHORT ANSWER TYPE QUESTIONS

1. Explain the structure and function of internal male reproductive system.
2. Describe the structure and function of uterus.
3. Draw a well label diagram of female reproductive system and explain its functions.

MULTIPLE CHOICE QUESTIONS

1. The external organs of female reproductive system are also known as:
   a. Genitalia
   b. Vulva
   c. Perineum
   d. Fundus
2. Which of the following comes under the functions of female reproductive system?
   a. Formation of ova
   b. Lactation
   c. Parturition
   d. All of the above
3. Which organ corresponds to the penis of male reproductive system?
   a. Clitoris
   b. Vestibule
   c. Labia majora
   d. Labia minora
4. Which of the following ligaments extends cervix and vagina to the side wall of pelvis?
   a. Broad ligaments
   b. Round ligaments
   c. Cardinal ligaments
   d. Uterosacral ligaments
5. Which organ lies in the pelvic cavity between the bladder and the rectum?
   a. Uterus
   b. Vagina
   c. Fallopian tubes
   d. Clitoris
6. Which is the part of external male reproductive system?
   a. Vas deferens
   b. Prostate gland
   c. Ejaculatory duct
   d. Penis

ANSWERS KEY

1. a
2. d
3. a
4. c
5. a
6. d

Chapter 12: Reproductive System

ATLAS

Identify and label the diagram.

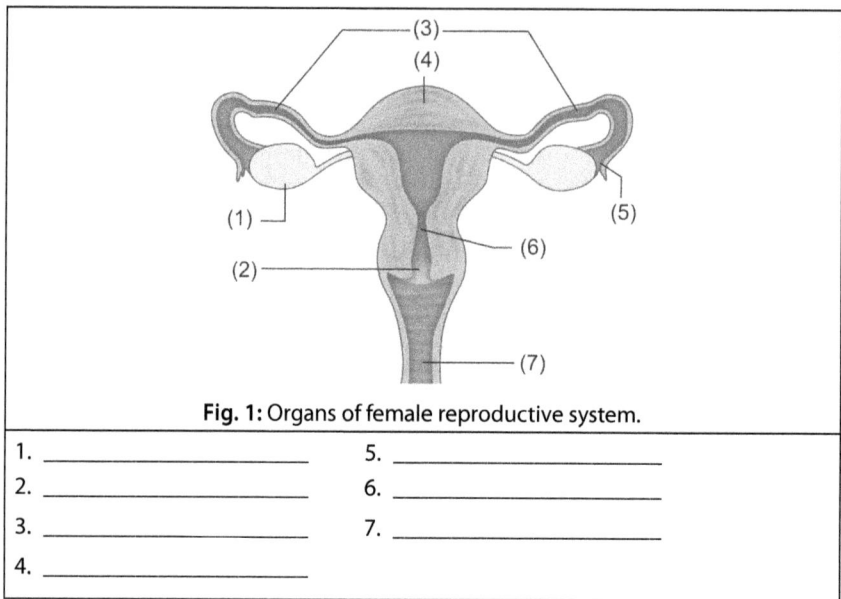

Fig. 1: Organs of female reproductive system.

1. _____
2. _____
3. _____
4. _____
5. _____
6. _____
7. _____

Index

Page numbers followed by f refer to figure and t refer to table.

A

Abdominal muscles 17
Acidophils 39
Acromegaly 127
Adenoids 68
Adipose cells 11
Adrenal cortex 124, 132, 133
Adrenal gland 121, 124, 125f, 130, 133
Adrenal insufficiency 128
Adrenal medulla 125, 132
Adrenaline 133
    hormone, functions of 126
Adrenocorticotrophic hormone 123, 124
Adrenocorticotropin 133
Adventitia 72
Agranular leukocytes 39
Aldosterone 125
Alveoli 64, 65f
Amenorrhea 133
Ampulla, fertilization occurs in 144
Anal canal 84
Anatomical planes 2f
Androgens 127, 133
Andropause 133
Anemia 41
    classification of 42t
Antibodies 41t
Antidiuretic hormone 123
Antigens 41t
Aorta 52, 55, 56
Aplastic anemia 42
Apnea 66
Appendicular skeleton 23, 26, 27f
Arachnoid mater 104
Arm, muscles of 17
Arteries 49, 55
Arterioles 49, 55
Atrioventricular bundle 53, 55
Atrioventricular node 52, 55
Auditory tube 29
Autonomic nervous system 108
Axial skeleton 22, 23, 24f
Axon 110

B

Basophil 39, 39f
Blood 34, 49
    cellular
        content of 35, 36f
        elements of 36
    clotting of 41
    coagulation 35, 41
        factors, nomenclature for 41
    composition of 34, 36f
    contains plasma 34
    different cells of 35f
    disorders of 41
    functions of 35
    group 40
    supply 73
Blood pressure 53, 55
    diastolic 54
    systolic 54
Blood vessel 49, 51, 55
    attached to heart 51f
    containing cells 34f
Body
    abdominopelvic cavity 4
    cavities in 3, 4f
    cranial cavity 3
    planes of 21, 22f
    thoracic cavity 3
    vertebral canal 3
Bones
    and muscles 16
    types of 29
Bowman's capsule 90
Brain 100, 100f, 111, 112
    lobes of 101, 102f, 111
    parts of 104f
Breast 145, 145f

Index

Bronchi 63, 63f
    disorders 63
Bursae 30

C

Cadaver 86
Calcitonin 133
Carbon dioxide 36
Cardiac cycle 53
Cardiac muscle 13, 16, 19, 20t
Cardiac output 53, 55
Cardiac sphincter 77
Cardiovascular system 34, 49
Cartilage 29, 68
    elastic 29
    hyaline 29
Cell 6
    alpha 126
    beta 126
    body 110
    mast 11
    pigment 11
    plasma 11
    structure of 6f
    transportation across 8
Central nervous system 100, 111, 112
Cerebellum 103
Cerebrospinal fluid 105, 112
Cerebrum 101, 101f, 112
Cervix 145
    cancer of 148
Choroid plexus 105
Chyme 85
Cilia 7
Clitoris 143
Clotting, disorders of 43
Collagen fibers 11
Columns of Bertini 89
Cones 119
Connective tissue 11
    cells of 11, 11f
    fibers of 11
    types of 12, 13f
Cortical nephron 92t
Corticosterone 124
Cortisol 133
Cortisone 124
Cranial nerves 108, 109t, 111, 112
    functions 109t
Cryptorchidism 147
Cushing's disease 128
Cushing's syndrome 129f
Cytoplasm 7
Cytosol 7

D

Dendrite 110, 112
Diabetes 130
Diencephalon 102, 103f
Digestion
    basic processes of 71
    physiology of 85
Digestive system 70
Distal convoluted tubule 91
Duct
    collecting 89
    ejaculatory 141
Dura mater 104
Dyspnea 66

E

Ear 29, 117f, 119
    audioception 117
    hearing 117
Early normoblast 37
Elastic fibers 11
Electrocardiogram 54
    components of 54f
Endocardium 56
Endocrine glands 121, 131t
Endocrine system 121, 121f
    disorders 127
    functions of 122
Endocrine tumors 129
Endoplasmic reticulum 8
Eosinophil 39, 39f
Epididymis 140
Epiglottis 29
Epispadias 148
Epithelium
    columnar 10
    cuboidal 10
    pseudostratified 10
    simple 9
    squamous 10
    stratified 10
    stratified squamous
        keratinized 10
        nonkeratinized 10
    tissue, types of 10f
    transitional 10
Erectile dysfunction 148
Erythroblastosis fetalis 41
Erythrocyte 36
    mature 37
Erythrocytosis 43
Erythropoiesis 37
Erythropoietin 133

Esophagus 70, 76, 76f
  functions of 76
Estradiol 133
Estrogen 127, 133
Excretion 88, 98
Excretory system 88
  disorders of 96
Exhalation 66
Eye 116f, 119
  ophthalmoception 116
  sight 116

F

Facial expression, muscles of 17
Fallopian tubes 144
Fertilization 149
Fibroblasts 11
Fibrocartilage 29
Fibrocytes 11
Filtration slits 90
Fimbria 144
Fissure 102, 102f
Flagella 7
Follicle stimulating hormone 146
Follicular phase 146
Foot muscles 17
Forearm, muscles of 17
Forebrain 100, 101

G

Gallbladder 81, 82f, 86
  functions of 81
  parts of 81
Gastroesophageal reflux disease 76
Gastrointestinal tract 70
  layers of 71, 71f
Genital organs
  external male 138f, 139
  internal male 140, 141f
Gigantism 129
Gingivitis 75
Glands 133
  location of 122
Glomerular filtration 92, 93f
  rate 98
Glomerulonephritis 97
Glossitis 75
Glucagon 133
Glucocorticoids 124
Glucose, synthesis of 126
Glycoproteins 40
Golgi complex 8
Gonadotrophic hormones 123

Gonads 132, 133
Grave's disease 129
Growth hormone 122
Gyri 102, 102f

H

Head skull, bones of 24, 24f
Heart 49, 56
  atrium 51
  conduction system of 52, 52f
  interior 50
  position of 50, 55
  sounds 53
  structure of 50f
  valves 51
Heart structure 50
  endocardium 50
  myocardium 50
  pericardium 50
Hemocytoblast 37
Hemodialysis 96
Hemoglobin 37
  functions of 38
  structure of 38f
Hemolysis 38
Hemolytic anemia 43
Hemophilia 43
Hilum 98
  renalis 89
Hindbrain 101, 103
Hip
  bone 29
  muscle 17
Homeostasis 4
Hormone 122, 133
Human anatomy, branches of 1
Human being, digestive system in 70f
Human body, movements of 1, 2f
Human excretory system 88
Human urinary system 89f
Hydrocortisone 124
Hyoid bone 25, 68
Hyperthyroidism 128
Hypoglycemia 129
Hypogonadism 130
Hypopituitarism 128
Hypothalamus 103, 133
Hypothyroidism 128

I

Infertility 148
Inhalation 66
Insulin 133

Interstitial cystitis 147
Iron deficiency anemia 42
Islets of Langerhans 126

J

Joints 29
   cartilaginous 29
   fibrous 29
   synovial 30
Juxtaglomerular apparatus, regulation involving 93
Juxtamedullary nephron 92t

K

Kidney 98
   function, regulation of 93, 96f
   location of 88
   longitudinal section of 89f
   retroperitoneal 88
   structure of 88

L

Labia majora 142
Labia minora 142
Large intestine 70, 83, 84f, 86
   ascending colon 84
   cecum 84
   descending colon 84
   functions of 84
   sigmoid colon 84
   transverse colon 84
Laryngopharynx 61
Larynx 62, 62f
   disorders 62
Leg muscles 17
Leukocytes 11, 38
Life, basic unit of 6
Ligaments 30
Limb radiography, positioning for 23f
Liver 80, 80f, 86, 96
   attachment of 81
   functions of 81
   lobes of 80
Locomotor system 16
Loop of Henle 91
Lower respiratory system 60
Lumbar tap 105
Lumber puncture 105
Lung 63, 64f, 96
   capacities 67
   disorders 64
   volumes 67

Luteal phase 147
Lymphocytes 39, 39f
Lysosomes 8

M

Macrophages 11
Malpighian body 90
Mastication, muscles of 17
Mechanical digestion 85
Mediastinum 69
Medulla oblongata 69, 103
Medullary pyramids 89
Medullary rhythmicity area 67
Megaloblastic anemia 42
Membrane repolarization 5
Meninges 103, 111
   membranes of 104f
Menstrual cycle 145, 146f
Mesenchymal cells 11
Microvilli 86
Midbrain 100
Mineralocorticoids 125
Mitochondria 8
Monocytes 39
   image of 40f
Mons pubis 142
Motor unit 18f
Mouth 72, 72f
   association with 72
   disorders of 75
Mucosa 71
Muscle contraction 18, 19f
   mechanism of 18
   types of 18
Muscle tissue, types of 16, 17f
Muscular system 16
   functions of 20
Muscular tissue 12
   types of 12, 13f
Muscularis 72
Musculoskeletal system 16
Myocardium 56

N

Nephron 94t, 98
   parts of 94f
   structure of 90, 91f
   types of 92
Nerve tissue 109
Nervous system 100, 111
   parasympathetic 110f
   sympathetic 110f
Nervous tissue 14

Index

Neuromuscular junction 18
Neuron, parts of 111f
Neutrophil 38, 39f
Noradrenaline hormone, functions of 126
Normoblast
   intermediate 37
   late 37
Nose 61f, 118
   olfalcoception 118
   smell 118
Nucleus 7, 7f
Nutrition 35, 70

O

Oral cavity 72f
Orbit, muscles of 17
Organelles 7
Organs in excretion, role of 96
Oropharynx 61
Orthopnea 66
Osmosis 9
Ossicle 25, 25f
Ovary 127, 127f, 130, 145, 148
Ovulation 149
Ovulatory phase 147
Oxygen and carbon dioxide, exchange of 67
Oxytocin 123

P

Pancreas 78, 79f, 126, 126f, 130, 132
   parts of 78
   types of 79
Pancreatic juice 79
   functions of 79
Papilla 86, 89
   circumvallate 73
   filiform 73
   foliate 73
   fungiform 73
   types of 73, 73f
Parasympathetic nervous system 109
Parathyroid gland 121, 124, 124f, 132
Pectoral girdle 27, 28f
Pelvic floor, muscles of 17
Pelvic girdle 27, 28f
Penis 139
Perineum 143
Peripheral nervous system 107, 107f, 111
   parts of 108f
Peristalsis 85, 86
Peritoneum 86
Pharyngitis 61

Pharynx 60, 61f, 70
   disorders 61
   muscles of 17
Physiology 2
   animal 3
   branches of 3
   cardiovascular 3
   cell 3
   comparative 3
   medical 3
   plant 3
Pia mater 104
Pineal gland 121, 127, 132
Pituitary gland 121, 122, 122f
   anterior 131
Plasma membrane 6
Platelets 40
   disorders of 43
Podocytes 90
Polycystic ovary syndrome 128
Polycythemia 43
Pons 68, 103
Proerythroblast 37
Progesterone 127
Prolactin 123
Prostate gland 140
Proximal convoluted tubule 90
Pulmonary arteries 52, 55, 56
Pulmonary respiration 65
Pulmonary veins 52, 55
Pulmonary ventilation 65
P-wave 54
Pyloric sphincter 78

Q

QRS complex 54

R

Rectum 84, 86
Red blood
   cells, matuaration of 37f
   corpuscles 36
Renal calculi 97
Renal calyx 89
Renal cortex 91
   outer 89
Renal failure 96
Renal medulla 89, 91
Renal pelvis 89
Renal pyramids 89
Renin angiotensin aldosterone system 5
Reproduction 149

Index

Reproductive organ 140
  external female 142, 142f
  internal female 143, 143f
Reproductive system 138
  disorders 147
  female 141
  function of
    female 143
    male 138
  male 138
  organ of female 145
Respiration 35
  alterations in 66
  chemoreceptor regulation of 68
  control of 67
  cortical influences on 68
  external 65, 67
  internal 65, 67
  physiology of 65, 66f
Respiratory center 5, 67
  regulation of 68
Respiratory system 60
  functions of 65
Respiratory zone 60
Reticular fiber 12, 12f
Reticulocyte 37
Rhesus system 40
Rib cage 25, 25f
Ribosomes 8
Rods 119
Rugae 86

S

Sacrum 29
Saliva
  composition of 75
  functions of 75
Salivary gland 74, 75f
Scapula 29
Scrotum 139
Semen 149
Seminal vesicles 140
Sense organs 114, 115, 115f, 116
  ears 115
  eyes 115
  nose 115
  skin 115
  tongue 115
Sensory organs 118
  proprioception system 118
  sensation receptors 118
Sensory receptors, types of 114
Serosa 72
Sex steroids 125

Shoulder, muscles of 17
Sinoatrial node 52, 55
Skeletal muscle 12, 16, 19, 20t
  structure of 17, 17f
Skeletal system 16, 22
  functions of 30
Skin 96, 118, 119
  tactioception 118
  touch 118
Skull bones 29
Slit pores 90
Small intestine 70, 82, 83f
  duodenum 82
  enzymes of 82
  functions of 83
  ileum 82
  jejunum 82
Smooth muscle 13, 16, 19, 20t
Special senses 114
Sphincter 86
Spinal cord 105, 106f, 111
Spinal nerves 108
Sternum 29
Stomach 70, 77, 77f
  curvatures of 77
  functions of 78
  layers arrangement in 78
  orifices of 77
  sphincters of 77
Stomatitis 75
Submucosa 72
Suprarenal gland 124, 130
Sympathetic nervous system 109
Synovial joint 30f

T

Teeth 74
  blood supply 74
  parts of 74, 74f
Tendon 19, 20f
Testes 127, 127f, 130, 139, 139f
Thalamus 103
Thigh muscle 17
Thrombocytes 40
Thymus 127, 130, 132
Thyroid gland 121, 123, 123f, 128f, 130
  functions of 124
Thyrotrophic hormone 123
Tissue 9, 65
  epithelial 9
Tongue 73, 117
  gustaoception 117
  muscles of 17
  taste 117

Index

Tonsillitis 61
Tonsils 68
Trachea 62
Transitional epithelium 89
Troponin 19, 19f
Tubular reabsorption, selective 92
Tubular secretion 93, 98
T-wave 54
Typical neuron, structure of 14f

U

Ultrafiltration 92
Upper respiratory system 60
Uremia 96
Ureter 89
Urethra 90, 141
Urinary bladder 89
Urinary tract, postrenal 89
Urine
    chemical composition of 93
    formation, mechanism of 92
    passage of 90
Urothelium 89
Uterine
    fibroids 147
    tube 144

Uterus 144
    parts of 144f

V

Vagina 144
Vas deferens 140
Vasopressin 123
Veins and venules 49, 55
Vena cava 51, 55, 56
    inferior 52, 55
    superior 51, 55
Ventricle 56, 104, 105f, 111
Vertebrae 29
Vertebral column 26, 26f

W

Wheezing 66
White blood cells 38
    classification of 38
    disorders of 43

EU GSPR Authorised Reprsentative
Logos Europe, 9 rue Nicolas Poussin
1700, La Rochelle, France
Phone: +33 (0) 6 67 93 73 78
E-mail: contact@logoseurope.eu